PILATES FOR BEGINNERS

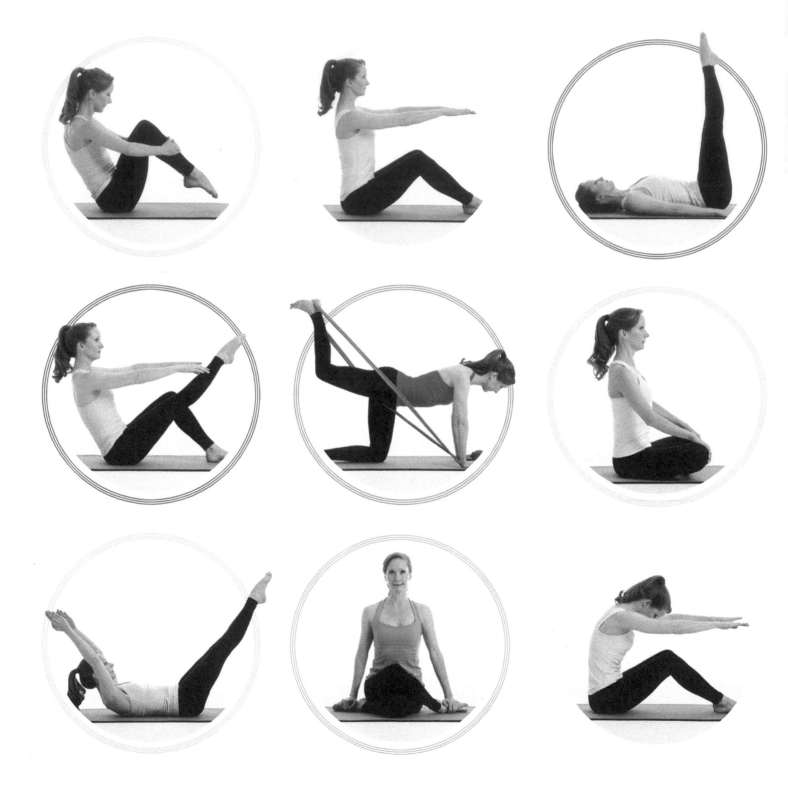

PILATES

FOR BEGINNERS

Katherine Corp & Kimberly Corp

Photography by Beth Bischoff

CORE PILATES
EXERCISES and
EASY SEQUENCES
to PRACTICE
at HOME

ALTHEA
PRESS

Designer: Merideth Harte
Editor: Meg Ilasco
Production Editor: Andrew Yackira
Photography © Beth Bischoff

ISBN: Print 978-1-64152-150-5 | eBook 978-1-64152-151-2

We dedicate this book to our family,
and all who supported us when we shifted
paths to the "road less traveled."

CONTENTS

INTRODUCTION

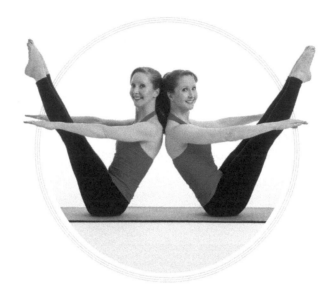

PILATES HAS LONG BEEN TOUTED for its ability to strengthen the core, sculpt long, lean muscles, and increase strength and flexibility. Professional dancers have used Pilates since the 1930s to maintain peak performance and prevent injury. In the late '80s, Pilates became popular among celebrities for increasing strength without muscle bulk. But because of its popularity among celebrities and dancers, a common misconception is that only people who are already fit can do Pilates.

This is absolutely not true! When practiced properly, Pilates can help anyone, of any age and fitness level, make lasting changes to their posture, core strength, flexibility, and overall fitness. Joseph Pilates originally called his system "Contrology"—the study of control—because he believed the exercises required complete control of mind, body, and spirit. Over time, "Contrology" became synonymous with "Pilates" as his disciples and students recommended the practice to others. Only in the 1980s, over 10 years after his death in 1967, did the name of his system transition to simply "Pilates." Pilates's direct disciples preserved his method diligently, and that practice is now referred to as "classical Pilates." Over time, Pilates practitioners have introduced slight modifications or adjustments to classical Pilates in order to incorporate modern knowledge of biomechanics (the anatomical way the body moves). As practitioners and teachers, we embrace Joseph Pilates's classical system, but have also recognized the need for modifications. Every *body* is different, so every *individual* may need to perform Pilates exercises with slight variations. You'll find many of our modified exercises throughout this book.

We first discovered Pilates while dancing on an international tour. We were in desperate need of a strengthening and maintenance program we could do in hotel rooms, backstage, or anywhere! Performing eight shows a week and sleeping on a bus or in a different hotel room every night wreaks havoc on the body.

But once we started practicing Pilates, our bodies felt stronger and healthier. Pilates improved our core strength and joint mobility very quickly, which kept us injury-free throughout our dancing careers—and even later, as Radio City Rockettes, dancing on a steel stage!

Following our dancing years, we continued practicing Pilates while earning graduate degrees in International Economic Policy at Columbia University. We soon realized we could combine our passion for movement and Pilates with our business skills, and the seed for our Manhattan studio, Pilates on Fifth, was planted. We opened it in the year 2000, and many years later, we're still thriving!

At our studio we've seen countless people transform their bodies and lives with Pilates. Many women turn to Pilates after childbirth, as it helps reestablish the brain-body connection to the abdominal muscles, especially after a C-section. One male client of ours (who admitted he was attending Pilates lessons just to appease his wife) was shocked to see how much his range of motion improved in spinal

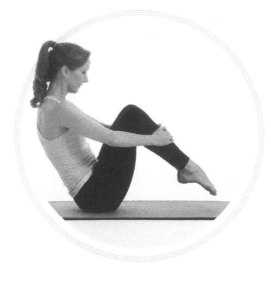

rotation and shoulder mobility, which greatly improved his golf game. An older female client still brags that she grew an inch in her 70s due to strengthening the deep postural muscles that support the spine. Clients routinely tell us that they are stronger now than they were 5 to 10 years ago, thanks to Pilates.

On a personal level, Pilates has helped us stay young in body and mind. We use Pilates daily to stay strong, flexible, and injury free, and it has helped us remain the size we were when we were dancing professionally. Pilates has given us the confidence in our bodies and in ourselves to meet life's challenges, and we're passionate about sharing the benefits with

as many people as possible. We wrote *Pilates for Beginners* to debunk the myth that Pilates is only for people who are already in great shape. In these pages, we share the fundamentals of Pilates exercises and teach strong technique out the gate to help anyone—even the absolute beginner—build a successful Pilates practice at home.

This book is structured in a way that will smoothly guide you on your Pilates journey. In Part One, Welcome to Pilates, we introduce the philosophy of Pilates and explain how to be mindful with your movements. If you're accustomed to fast-paced cardio like running or spinning, you may not have experience *thinking* about the quality of each and every move, so we will help you get into the right mind-set. We then introduce our Guiding Principles of Pilates—Centering, Concentration, Control, Precision, Breath, and Flow—which you'll incorporate into every practice. From there, we include a list of words and terms to help you follow the Pilates exercises in this book and beyond. We explain everything you'll need to get started, as well as modifications for pain and injuries.

Part Two is when you get moving. This section presents 50 exercises, including warm-ups, cooldowns, and bonus strengthening exercises. In the Introductory Program, you mobilize the spine in all directions and build core strength and body awareness with deliberate, mindful movements. The Introductory Program is the ultimate foundation. Just as you would not construct a building of multiple stories without first establishing a firm, strong foundation, you should resist moving on to Level 1 before mastering the exercises in the introductory section. Level 1 builds on the Introductory Program with full versions of Pilates exercises, which require more strength, range of motion, and control. By this time, you'll have a strong understanding of your own body, specifically which exercises you can do and which you might need to modify. Finally, Level 2 presents exercises that require even more strength, spinal mobility, flexibility, and control. As with the Level 1 Program, you'll likely find that certain types of exercises are easier than others, so be patient with yourself and modify as necessary.

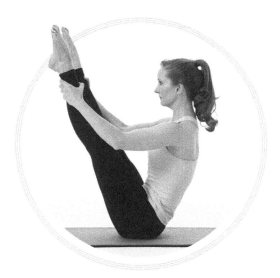

In the end, true fitness isn't just about burning calories. It's about a healthy spine, healthy joints, and the freedom to move through life with ease and without injury. Pilates has kept us just as active in our 40s as we were in our 20s, and we know that Pilates can do the same for you! Pilates will not only make you stronger, but also (and more importantly) keep your body supple and mobile, adding more life to your years. We're excited to accompany you on your Pilates journey.

Now let's get started!

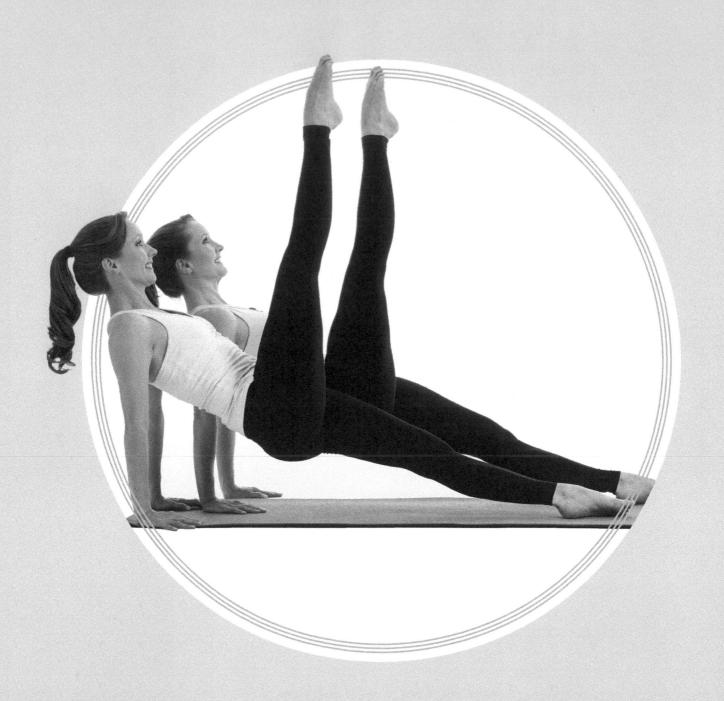

PART ONE

WELCOME TO PILATES

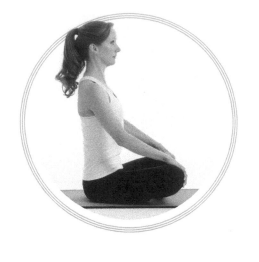

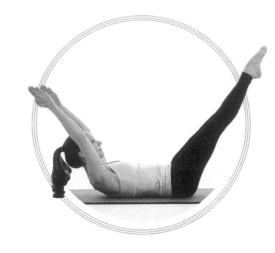

CHAPTER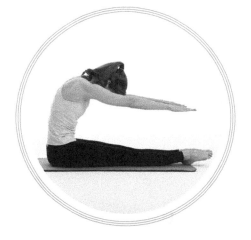

1

PILATES 101

WHEN YOU FIRST SEE PILATES IN ACTION, it can appear to be no different than the typical abdominal exercises. But it's so much more! Joseph Pilates designed each exercise carefully with a specific intent. He believed you should focus your mind fully on the intent and execution of the movement. The system is designed around his belief that a strong core, or "powerhouse," is the foundation of all efficient movement.

PILATES PHILOSOPHY

Joseph Pilates's beliefs on health and wellness were inspired by the ancient Greek and Roman philosophies of physical and mental well-being. Pilates adopted the Roman motto *mens sana in corpore sano*, which translates to "a sane mind in a sound body." He believed the only path to true happiness is the strengthening of the mind and body simultaneously, and he identified various techniques to help people get there.

Visualization to Engage Your Mind and Body

Once considered to be a mystical or new age belief, visualization—the act of forming mental images to aid in movement execution—has been scientifically proven to enhance athletic performance.

Broadly speaking, there are two types of visualizations that can enhance your Pilates experience: One uses imagery and the other uses anatomy. For instance, to achieve flat abdominal muscles and the concept of "drawing in," we might say to our students, "Pull your belly button to your spine." This is an anatomical visualization. Or we could say, "Imagine you're squeezing an orange between your belly button and your spine," which is an image-based visualization.

Because not all visualizations work for each individual, we include both imagery-based and anatomy-based visualizations in this book. We do this to help you concentrate on the movement you are performing. By focusing on the muscle being targeted and the proper physical execution of the exercise, visualizations engage the mind and the muscles, leading to better overall results.

Focusing on Your Powerhouse

Joseph Pilates coined the word "powerhouse" to describe the lower two-thirds of your torso. This runs from the base of your chest (the pectoral muscles) to the crease of your hips, continuing down to the base of your pelvis. In the powerhouse are your four abdominal muscles: your lower back muscles, the deep muscles surrounding your spine, your diaphragm, and the muscles of your pelvic floor. The word is interchangeable with the mainstream term "core," but remember that both terms comprise much more than just "the abs"!

Pilates believed that the combination of a strong powerhouse, a supple spine, and breath coordinated with action is the foundation for all healthy movement. According to Pilates, range of motion is always secondary to abdominal control and proper technique. Every movement—whether you're pitching a ball or practicing Pilates—generates from a strong center. So be sure to focus on the powerhouse during the exercises in this book. With each exercise, activate your powerhouse before you begin, and make sure it stays engaged during the entire movement. This will become automatic with time, but don't get discouraged if at first you must consciously think of activating and reengaging the powerhouse. Once you get in the habit, you'll begin to feel the difference in how you move both on and off the mat.

Balancing Strength, Flexibility, and Spinal Movements

Joseph Pilates began his 1945 book, *Return to Life Through Contrology*, with a chapter entitled "Civilization Impairs Physical Fitness." It laments how the hectic 1940s lifestyle was wreaking havoc on modern civilization's posture. Imagine if he had lived to see the world of smartphones, texting, laptops, and tablets! Sadly, we are far more sedentary today than people were during Pilates's lifetime. This means his goal to improve posture through exercise is even more important today.

Joseph Pilates designed his signature system using a balance of strength and flexibility in order to correct bad habits and restore the body to its natural, upright carriage. Pilates also balanced targeting small, deeper muscles along with larger, superficial muscles, which leads to increased total body strength.

Far ahead of his time, Joseph Pilates dismissed the adage "you're only as old as you feel" and instead believed that you're only as old as your spine. Therefore, every Pilates exercise involves specific spinal movements, even if the motion is as subtle as stabilizing the spine against the movement of the limbs. Given the increasingly sedentary nature of society, and the fact that people spend too much time rounded over desks and phones, we need to incorporate even more spinal movements into our Pilates practice today. To balance the number of forward-bending (flexion) exercises in Joseph Pilates's original repertoire, we've added a few more exercises that involve back bending (extension), side bending, and rotation. These additional exercises are commonly practiced in Pilates studios today.

WHAT PILATES CAN BRING TO YOUR LIFE

Pilates can provide physical and mental benefits to anyone who practices it. You're never too old, too out of shape, or too busy to start reaping the benefits of Pilates. The amazing benefits we've personally experienced and been honored to observe in our clients include:

Increased core strength: Pilates strengthens the deep muscles surrounding your spine, as well as your abdominal and back muscles. This leads to more power in simple daily tasks such as lifting, changing direction quickly, or even climbing stairs. On top of that, increased core strength aids in injury prevention: Your spine is bolstered for the unexpected, whether it's a slip, a fall, or a surprise impact.

Increased flexibility: Pilates increases flexibility by moving the spine and limbs through all ranges of motion. Most of us think about flexibility in terms of extremes (like doing splits), but functional flexibility is really about simple actions like getting up and down off the floor, getting in and out of a chair without using your arms, stepping in and out of the bathtub, washing your hair comfortably, and even taking long strides to keep up with your kids or friends. The amount of flexibility we have in our spines and muscles determines our freedom of motion as we get older.

Improved posture: Because Pilates focuses on proper alignment in every exercise, your posture quickly improves. The aesthetic benefits of good posture are obvious: You look taller, more confident, and usually more slender as well. However, beyond aesthetics, improved posture has been linked to better breathing, reduced back pain, and a decrease in chronic headaches, to name a few benefits.

Freedom in the spine and joints: Pilates increases mobility of the spine and joints,

THE MAN BEHIND THE MOVEMENT

Joseph Pilates embarked on a path of health and fitness at a young age to overcome his own childhood sicknesses. Born in Germany in 1880 just outside of Dusseldorf, Pilates suffered from asthma, rickets, and rheumatic fever. To improve his health, he practiced diving, skiing, bodybuilding, and gymnastics to great success. At age 14, Pilates even posed as a model for anatomy charts.

In 1914, during the outbreak of World War I, Pilates was interned with other German nationals in England. During his internment, he began developing a system of exercises he called "Contrology" (the study of control), which is known today as "Pilates." To help the less mobile of his fellow internees build strength and improve their fitness, he used simple bedsprings to design the prototypes of what would go on to become his mass-produced Pilates equipment.

Pilates immigrated to New York City in 1926 and joined a boxers' training gym in a building that also housed dance schools and rehearsal spaces. Pilates quickly grew a reputation for helping performers with injuries, and word of his method spread quickly through New York City's dance scene and high society. Despite having great success locally, Pilates endeavored to see his work accepted by the medical community—to no avail. However, as his early students began moving away from New York, the public's awareness of Pilates's exercises and their benefits expanded.

Sadly, a 1966 fire at his studio seems to have led to his death in October of 1967 at the age of 87. Thankfully, many of his students continued his work, establishing Pilates studios and practices throughout the country. Decades ahead of its time, Pilates's system of exercises is now widely considered one of the best mind-body disciplines available.

which allows you to move with more freedom of motion. As we age, the natural range of motion in our spine and joints decreases unless we take deliberate action to keep them mobile. Pilates exercises can keep us moving through our functional range of motion throughout our lives.

Balanced muscle development: Pilates designed his exercises to balance muscular development between large and small muscles, deep and superficial muscles, and the muscles surrounding a joint. When the right muscle is working in the right amount of intensity at the right time, muscles develop uniformly without certain muscle groups becoming overdeveloped at the expense of others. And since Pilates increases strength and flexibility simultaneously, a practitioner of Pilates achieves long, strong muscles without muscle bulk.

Harmony of movement: Typical exercises in a gym isolate one muscle group at a time: the biceps, the triceps, the glutes, or the knee extensors. However, everyday actions require that our muscles work together—in harmony—to produce a

movement. Because Pilates exercises never isolate one muscle group, the body and the mind are trained to work as one cohesive unit.

Improved awareness: By focusing on alignment and technique, Pilates helps you become aware of your body and carriage at all times. The number one comment we receive from our clients is that Pilates has made them more mindful of how they carry themselves, even when they are outside of the studio. This awareness encompasses not only exercise endeavors but also simple tasks such as sitting properly, standing properly, and walking more upright.

Increased vitality: The stress of daily life coupled with suboptimal posture often leaves us susceptible to shallow breathing. Pilates exercises encourage deep, mindful breathing, which in turn circulates more oxygen to the brain and thus increases vitality.

Greater sense of calm: Pilates involves focusing on the breath, technique, and alignment, and this practice helps quiet the mind and bring more focus and calmness to your life.

GUIDING PRINCIPLES

In his books, Joseph Pilates cites whole-body health, whole-body commitment, and breath as the three guiding principles of his work. Since then, his disciples have derived additional principles based on his writings and teachings. The Guiding Principles here include Pilates's original principles as well as the principles incorporated into the Pilates vernacular over the years. The descriptions are true to Pilates's intent while also reflecting our own experience teaching many different clients over the years.

Centering: Centering has both physical and mental applications. It means focusing on the core and powerhouse in every exercise, which will enhance your quality of movement (since all movements of the body are improved by a strong center). It also means drawing your attention to your body and the specific muscles working in each moment. The concept of "centering" also means that you stay focused on yourself and do not compete with or compare yourself to others. Every *body* is different with a different genetic makeup and different life experiences. Center your thoughts on *you* and focus only on *your* body's needs.

Concentration: Joseph Pilates believed that full mental concentration was necessary to achieve the intended results of his system. If you practice Pilates and allow your thoughts to wander to a grocery list, tomorrow's conference call, upcoming weekend obligations, or an awkward conversation from yesterday, then—according to Joseph Pilates—this is *not* Pilates! Better results will be gained by fully concentrating on the specific movement. If you find that concentrating is difficult at first, try focusing on your breathing while doing the movement. This can help quiet the mind and bring attention to your center.

Control: Because Pilates exercises involve specific movements coordinated with the breath, a great deal of physical and mental control is required to perform the exercises as they were designed. Moving with controlled, deliberate motions challenges the body and mind in ways that other exercise does not. In fact, when each exercise is performed with the maximum amount of physical and mental control, only a few repetitions are necessary to reap the benefits. Learning to control your breath and movements has a positive impact on other aspects of life as well. More specifically, studies show that breath control has a profound impact on relaxation and stress relief.

Precision: Joseph Pilates designed his exercises with specific directions for body placement, movement sequencing, and breath. Intent on creating a balanced system of exercise for the whole body, Pilates chose every movement and breath for a reason. So when you practice Pilates with attention to detail, the muscles of the body work in concert to perform the task. Learning the precise technique and execution of the exercises from the start of your Pilates journey is essential to your success.

Breath: Deep breathing increases the body's oxygen intake and stimulates circulation. Pilates assigned specific breath patterns to each exercise. He believed that coordinating the breath with the movement leads to greater mental and physical benefits. At first, you may have trouble remembering when and how to breathe. That's okay. It's common for beginners to hold their breath when they think they're wrong, but please don't do this! As you practice Pilates, breathe fully, even if your breath doesn't initially match the instructions. Don't worry or stress about it. Over time, the breath coordination will become natural and automatic.

Flow: The flow of Pilates is experienced in three ways. First, the choreography of each exercise involves many muscle groups, which rhythmically contract and release to create fluid movement. After moving in one direction, the exercise takes you smoothly in another direction. Second, once the exercises are learned, they can be performed in sequence to flow seamlessly from one exercise to the next. Finally, movements in Pilates are never intended to be jerky or abrupt. Instead, they flow as if moving through water. This quality of movement transfers to other activities and can help you achieve more poise and grace in your carriage and gait. Keep in mind, however, that technique, precision, breath, and control always come before the principle of flow.

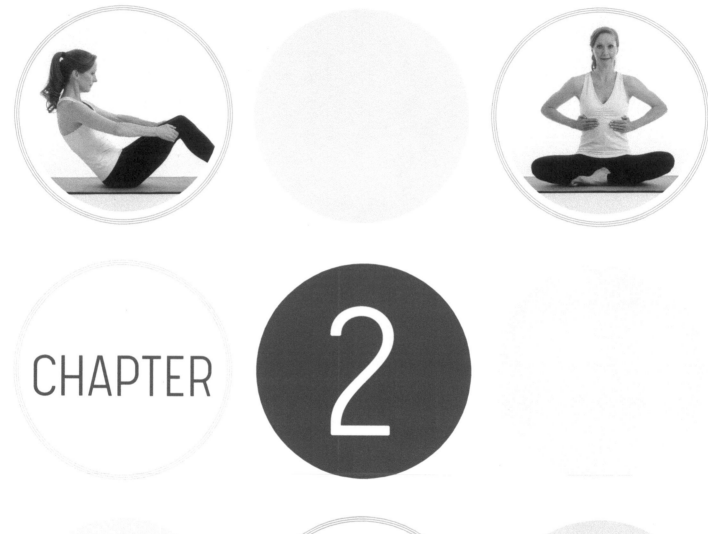

CHAPTER 2

PREPARING FOR THE MAT

PILATES IS MORE THAN EXERCISE—it's a healthy lifestyle choice that requires a commitment. In this chapter, we guide you through the process of getting started, including what to wear, how to create a comfortable workout space, how to choose a mat, and more. We also set you up for success in understanding and memorizing the exercises, transitions, and—most importantly—the language of Pilates.

MAKE A COMMITMENT TO PILATES

We know you're busy. We totally get it! But it's easier than you think to fit Pilates into your busy schedule. Consistency is the key to success, so all we're asking as you begin is that you commit to practicing for 20 to 30 minutes a day, four to five times per week.

Studies show that people who commit to a morning exercise regime are much more likely to stick to it. We suggest setting your alarm 30 minutes earlier than you usually do, with the intent of practicing Pilates. If a morning workout isn't possible, carve out four to five time slots each week that you can dedicate to Pilates.

Do your best to stick with this schedule for two to three months. You'll likely find that after three months, your 20- to 30-minute sessions naturally turn into 30- to 40-minute sessions, which is great! We encourage you to build your practice as it becomes available.

You may want to block off time in your calendar so there are no scheduling conflicts, and to help you avoid procrastination. Make an appointment with yourself, and keep it. A Pilates journal is a great way to monitor your progress and hold yourself accountable.

Remember, Pilates is a marathon, not a sprint. Dedication and consistency are essential.

WHAT YOU NEED TO BEGIN

Pilates is a convenient and affordable way to begin exercising. You don't need fancy equipment, and all the moves can be executed at home in a relatively small space. Here are some essentials to consider before you get started.

What to Wear

Choose comfortable clothing that allows for a wide range of movement. You don't need any fancy fitness wear, but if that motivates you, then go for it! Choose clothing that doesn't restrict your movement in any way and allows heat to escape. Loose clothing may be more comfortable, but avoid items that are so baggy the seams start to twist or you find yourself constantly adjusting your clothing.

We prefer form-fitting workout wear in a blend of Supplex, Lycra, nylon, and spandex. The material should breathe, have moisture-wicking attributes, and not be so tight that your range of motion is inhibited.

As Pilates exercises work on movement of the foot and ankle in addition to the whole body, footwear isn't needed. If you're practicing at home, barefoot is great. You can also wear socks with treads on the bottom, which provide traction to execute the exercises.

Choosing a Mat

When selecting a Pilates mat, choose one that's approximately 6 feet long, 2 feet wide, and ¼ to ½ inch thick. While you can use a yoga mat, they are typically much thinner (less than ⅛ inch thick), and therefore don't provide the same level of comfort needed to perform certain Pilates exercises. If you're exercising on carpet, you may not need a mat (but you may still want one, as carpet fibers can get itchy and stick to your clothing or hair). If you have allergies, then you may opt for a bamboo mat.

Making Space

When creating a space for your Pilates practice, choose an area that you find quiet and calming. Make sure your space is clear of furniture and obstacles. When gauging the size of the space, be mindful of the fact that Pilates requires room for your arms and legs to move in all directions. While it can be extremely soothing to make a space of your own for your practice, we admit that we've been known to exercise in front of the TV while someone's watching golf. It's really a matter of personal preference. And don't forget your pets! Your furry friend might think you're playing, and you don't want to inadvertently kick or roll on Fido or Kitty while practicing your Pilates.

WHAT TO EXPECT

Pilates is a comprehensive system with specific choreography of movement and breath for each exercise. As you practice, it's important to remember the choreography of each exercise and stay mindful of the coordination of breath and movement.

Memorization

The first step of Pilates is learning and memorizing the choreography for each exercise. However, rather than sitting down with this book and memorizing with your brain alone, we recommend that you do the exercises as you memorize so that you learn with your body and your brain. You don't need to master each individual exercise before moving on to the next, but we do recommend that you master all of the exercises in each section before moving on to the next level.

Fluid Transitions

Keeping with the concept of mindfulness is the theme of fluid transitions. Rather than executing individual exercises, you want to move with purpose from one exercise to the next. In other words, when you complete an exercise, try to maintain your form, posture, and intent before fluidly moving into the next. As you work through the programs in this book, stay mindful of your body during all transitions: Your breathing should remain fluid and calm, and movements should be deliberate and controlled.

LEARN THE LANGUAGE

Even if you're an avid exerciser, if you jump into a Pilates class without any briefing, you'll hear some unfamiliar terms. We want to provide you with the Pilates vocabulary you need to get the most out of your practice. All Pilates terms are based on movement principles. As you grow accustomed to pairing the terms with the movements, they'll become second nature. The common cues and terms below are used throughout this book, but this is by no means an exclusive list.

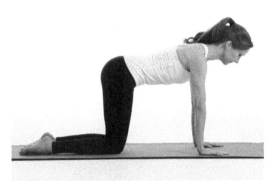 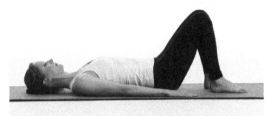

All fours: A common starting position in Pilates, this is the cue to get onto your hands and knees ("all fours") with your wrists directly under your shoulders and your knees under your hips. Your pelvis and spine should be neutral and hips flexed to 90 degrees. Pull your shoulders down and draw your belly button to your spine.

Chin to chest: With Pilates exercises that start by lying on your back, the first cue before lifting your head and shoulders off the mat will usually be "chin to chest." This is meant to prompt a slight tilt of the chin, just enough to protect your neck—there's no need to jam your chin down into your chest.

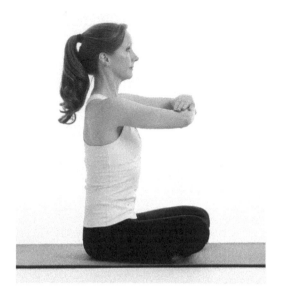

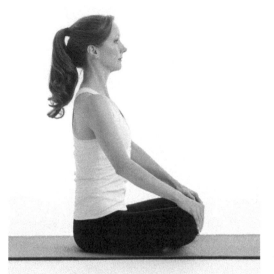

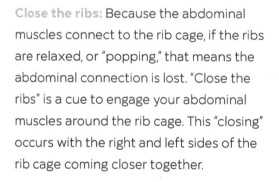

Close the ribs: Because the abdominal muscles connect to the rib cage, if the ribs are relaxed, or "popping," that means the abdominal connection is lost. "Close the ribs" is a cue to engage your abdominal muscles around the rib cage. This "closing" occurs with the right and left sides of the rib cage coming closer together.

Ears back: When standing or sitting in Pilates, proper head placement entails positioning the center of your ear over the center of your shoulder. Most of us tend to tilt our heads forward past our shoulders (especially when leaning over a screen!), so the cue "ears back" is helpful in assuming proper alignment.

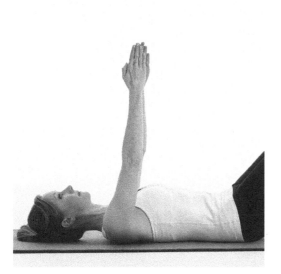

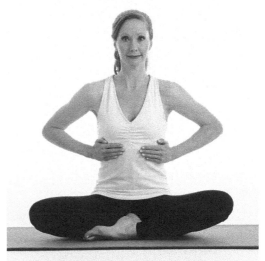

Imprint position: When performing certain Pilates exercises on your back, engaging the abdominal muscles makes the difference between getting stronger and getting injured. The term "imprint" is often used to cue moving the hip bones closer to the rib cage and pressing the lower back into the mat (leaving an "imprint"). However, for certain body types, this is difficult or even impossible to achieve. Actually imprinting your spine is not vital. What's important is creating a strong abdominal connection by closing the distance between the ribs and the hips.

Lateral breathing: This refers to breathing into the sides and back of the lungs as opposed to allowing the chest to elevate and the belly to inflate, as is common in yoga. This is the preferred breathing technique for Pilates.

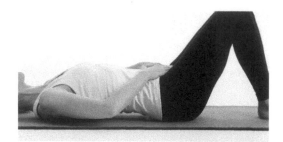

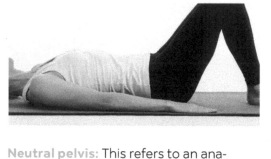

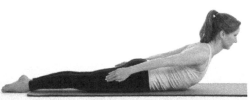

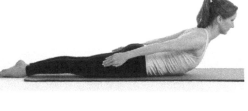

Lengthen: The image of lengthening is used extensively in Pilates, whether to "lengthen the back of your neck" or "lengthen your spine." This is an *image*, meaning that no change in the length of bones or muscles will actually occur. But cues to lengthen can help you tap in to the proper muscles to improve overall posture and form.

Neutral pelvis: This refers to an anatomical state when the pelvis is level in both the horizontal and vertical planes. When standing, imagine your pelvis as a basin of water. You want the water in the basin to be level and balanced so that it cannot spill out the front or back. If you tilt your pelvis forward, lowering your hip bones toward the floor, then the water would spill out the front. If you tuck your tailbone under too much, lifting the hip bones, water would spill out the back. When lying on the mat, make sure that the triangle created by your hip bones and pubic bone is parallel to the floor, and that you feel your tailbone on the mat (not lifted).

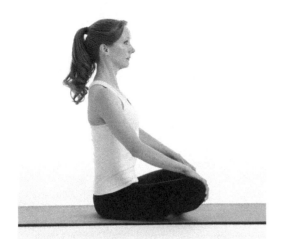
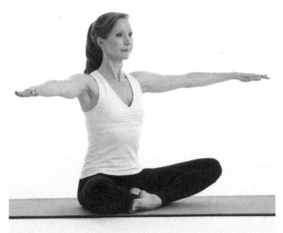

Neutral spine: Contrary to popular belief, the spine is not meant to be perfectly straight. The spine has three natural curves, which are important for proper movement of the spine and shock absorption in the body. The three curves occur in the neck region (cervical spine), the rib cage region (thoracic spine), and the lower back (lumbar spine). The spine in the neck region naturally curves forward, the spine in the rib cage region naturally curves toward the rear, and the spine in the lower back naturally curves forward again. The spine is considered "neutral" when these natural curves are present and not exaggerated (as they are when you are sitting hunched over).

Open your chest: Most activities in today's world bring our shoulders and head forward, whether we're seated at a desk, playing on our smartphones, or driving. The image of opening the chest or collarbone helps combat this natural tendency to hunch over and activates the muscles that create a better, more upright posture.

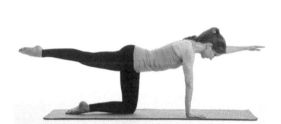

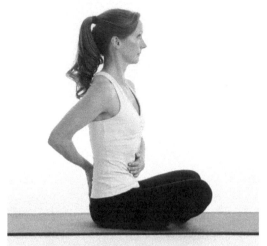

Opposition: This term applies to several concepts. Stability versus mobility, control versus release, "close the ribs but open the chest"—these are all examples of the oppositions we work with in Pilates. Muscles also move in opposition: When a muscle contracts, the opposing muscle lengthens. Even the image of lengthening involves a sense of opposition because we're envisioning a pull from opposite ends of the spine to create the length. As a core concept, this is a term you'll hear regularly in Pilates.

Pull your belly button to your spine: Pulling your belly button to your spine, almost as if you're putting on a corset or zipping up a tight pair of jeans, activates the deepest abdominal muscles, the transversus abdominis. True to its name, this muscle transverses the abdomen, with the fibers running horizontally and connecting to the fascia in the back. Because the transversus abdominis lies the closest to the spine, it plays more of a role in protecting the spine than the other three abdominal muscles. When you pull your belly button to your spine, you're both flattening the abs and creating amazing protection for the spine.

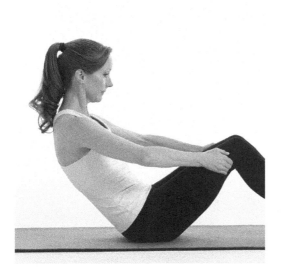 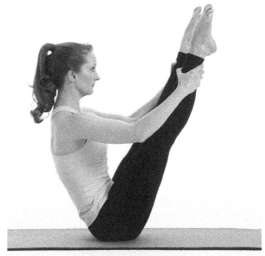

Scoop your belly/C-curve: These cues are two sides of the same coin. When you focus on scooping the belly, your spine will naturally move into a C-curve, and if you think of creating a C-curve in your spine, you will naturally engage your abdominal muscles (i.e., scoop your belly). Just like the cue to pull the belly button to your spine, scooping the belly engages the deepest layer of the abs to flatten the abs and protect your spine and lower back.

Stabilize: The ability to stabilize your joints effectively allows you to isolate and target specific muscle groups for functional training, as well as injury prevention. Pilates exercises promote dynamic stabilization so the spine and joints are protected while the limbs can move freely.

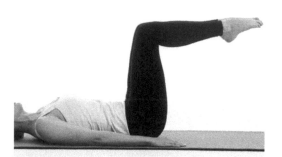

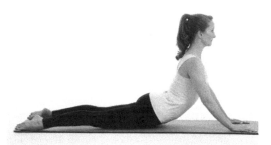

Tabletop position: This is a common starting position in which the hips and the knees are flexed at 90 degrees with the shins parallel to the floor, creating a "tabletop."

Threshold: Threshold is the point at which proper form can no longer be maintained. For example, in the image above for Swan Dive, Modified (page 71), if abdominal support cannot be maintained, the stress will go into the lower back. You've met threshold if you start feeling this in the back.

Pilates emphasizes ideal form in each and every exercise, and calls for an exercise to be stopped if proper form cannot be maintained. The suggested repetitions for each exercise are guidelines only and should be abandoned if form is compromised.

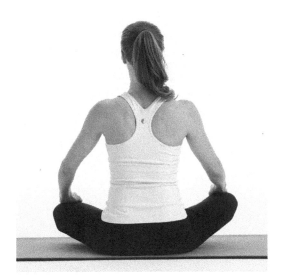

Wings down: "Wings" refers to the scapulas (shoulder blades), and the cue "wings down" is the act of pulling down the shoulder blades in order to stabilize the shoulder joints. The shoulder is a difficult joint to stabilize because it's designed for wide ranges of motion, such as those required in tennis, gymnastics, or swimming. Mindfully pulling down your "wings" for certain Pilates exercises is essential for building strength and preventing injury.

HOW TO USE THIS BOOK

When starting Pilates, allow yourself to *be* a beginner. Just as you would not achieve a black belt after your first martial arts class, you shouldn't expect instant mastery of Pilates! The book is organized to work through as you progressively build your strength, flexibility, balance, and endurance. While you may be tempted to jump ahead, we strongly recommend spending time with each section and only progressing to the next level when you are ready in body and mind.

Warm-Ups and Cooldowns

Warm-up exercises serve to prepare both the body and the mind for your Pilates practice. In addition to increasing core body temperature and gently mobilizing the spine, the warm-up allows you to let go of distracting thoughts and focus on yourself and your movements. The exercises activate the key muscle groups that should be engaged when practicing Pilates, and the sequence serves to mobilize the spine and stabilize the core.

In contrast, cooldown exercises bring your body temperature back down, while letting you relax in the success of your workout. The cooldown provides the perfect time to feel and appreciate the work you're putting into your health and well-being. We've chosen relaxing hip stretches for the cooldown, as many Pilates exercises work the muscles around the hips, mainly the hip flexors, in addition to the abs. This book has two hip stretches, one for the hip flexors at the front of the hip and another for the muscles on the side of the hip.

Introductory Program

Whether you're a fitness fanatic or a comfy couch potato, if you are new to Pilates, begin with this Introductory Program. Success in any endeavor requires the proper foundation, and this program was created to teach the techniques and fundamentals of Pilates that are necessary to reap the most benefits. Here we focus specifically on exercises that build strength in the abs and core. These exercises are straightforward, emphasizing proper posture and form as opposed to complexity of movement.

EXERCISE KEY

Each exercise in the book includes a quick guide of the following key components to help you study and remember each movement.

Focus: The goal of the exercise so you can focus your attention appropriately.

Repetitions: The number of times an exercise should be repeated with proper form and technique.

Visualization: Any imagery that may be useful in executing the exercise correctly.

Precautions: Certain conditions or injuries, if any, that dictate that an exercise should be avoided completely.

Dos and Don'ts: A quick, at-a-glance list of things you want to be sure you do for the exercise, and, perhaps more importantly, things you definitely do NOT want to do.

Assuming you're able to practice for 20 to 30 minutes a day four to five times per week, mastery of this program should take between two and three weeks. At the end of the section, you'll find a self-assessment questionnaire to help you understand the unique needs of your body and determine if you're ready to move to the next level.

Level 1 Program

Level 1 builds upon the foundations created in the Introductory Program while focusing on building strength and refining your Pilates technique. The moves in this program are more difficult in terms of strength, technique, and choreography. We recommend spending three to four weeks mastering the Level 1 Program. We also provide a Level 1 self-assessment questionnaire to track your progress and determine if you're ready to move to Level 2.

Level 2 Program

With the Level 2 Program, we delve more deeply into the full repertoire created by Joseph Pilates, adding greater challenges to strength and coordination. If the exercises feel too challenging, we provide modifications or "stepping stones" so you can progress safely without sacrificing technique. Expect to stick with Level 2 for four to five weeks, as these exercises are more demanding in terms of both strength and coordination. A self-assessment questionnaire at the end of the program will help you determine if you've mastered Level 2.

At the end of Level 2, we recommend maintaining a Pilates regimen of 20 to 30 minutes a day two to three times a week. All of the exercises in this book are sufficient for maintaining a healthy spine, core strength, and standard ranges of joint motion. However, if you'd like to take your Pilates practice further, you can either find a certified instructor near you, or visit an online video site such as PilatesOnFifthOnline.com to continue to build your Pilates prowess.

MODIFICATIONS FOR PAIN & INJURIES

Pilates should always make you feel better and stronger. Modifications are important in achieving this goal. Don't shy away from them. When either pain or an injury is present, MODIFY! Here are some simple modifications for you to consider as you work through the exercises. If you still experience pain after modifying and reducing the range of motion, then avoid the exercise altogether. And if you are injured, always get a doctor's clearance before doing Pilates.

Back: It may be necessary to limit the range of motion of certain exercises so that all movement is pain free in your back. If you feel discomfort in a neutral spine, adjusting to an imprint or supported position may alleviate the discomfort. If you're lying on your stomach, then a small cushion under the hip bones can be used to relax the back.

Knees: For knee problems, reduce the degree to which you bend your knee, and work only within your pain-free range of motion. Avoid start positions that cause pain (e.g., on all fours).

Hips: Hip discomfort in seated exercises is usually the result of tightness in the hip flexors. A cushion or pillow underneath the sit bones will help alleviate the pain.

Neck: If your head doesn't comfortably reach the ground when lying on your back, then place a pillow or cushion under your head that's high enough to bring your spine into a neutral position.

Shoulders: Reducing the range of motion of an exercise can alleviate shoulder pain that stems from either an injury or long term, chronic discomfort.

Wrists: By rolling up the edge of your mat and placing the heel of your hand on the rolled edge, you can reduce the angle of the wrist joint and alleviate discomfort.

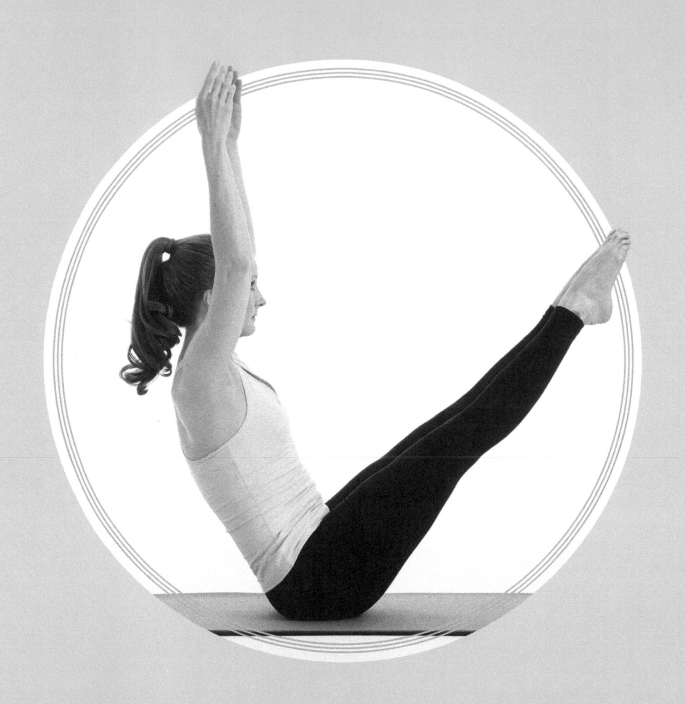

PART TWO

ON THE MAT

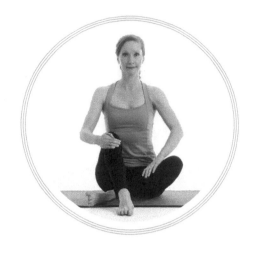

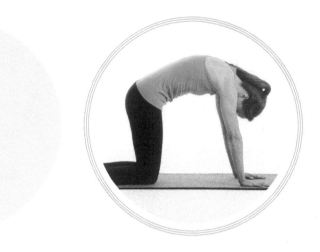

CHAPTER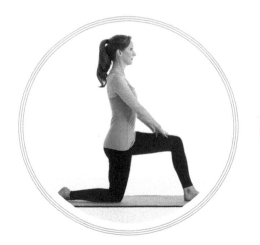

3

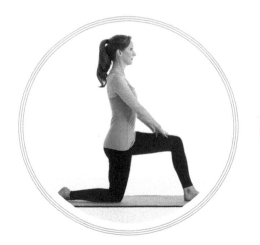

WARM-UPS & COOLDOWNS

WARM-UP EXERCISES CENTER THE BODY AND MIND, connecting you to your powerhouse and establishing the mindfulness needed to get the most out of your Pilates practice. To prepare the body, the warm-up activates important muscle groups, mobilizes the spine gently, and begins to generate heat in the body. To prepare the mind, the exercises enable you to let go of distractions and focus on yourself and the movements. Don't skip your warm-up! The cooldown is equally important. Our cooldown exercises include gentle hip stretches for the muscles at the front and sides of the hips, and these stretches should be performed slowly while focusing on breathing and centering your mind. These stretches will release any muscles that were active during your Pilates practice.

CAT STRETCH (WARM-UP)

The Cat Stretch mobilizes the spine. In this exercise, you mindfully coordinate the breath with curling and arching (flexing and extending) the spine. The Cat Stretch also helps build awareness of your spinal positions in space.

FOCUS: Mobilize the spine through curling and arching (flexing and extending) and coordinate the breath with each movement.

REPETITIONS: 3 to 5

VISUALIZATION: Imagine pushing the floor away as you hollow out your abs and lift your rib cage to the ceiling. Then keep the abs pulled to the spine as you lift the head and tailbone and release the rib cage toward the mat.

PRECAUTIONS: If you have knee discomfort or injuries, you may need to kneel on cushions or a blanket, or perform this exercise standing with your hands on a chair. If you have lower-back issues, be careful to limit the movement to your pain-free range of motion.

1. Assume an all-fours position (page 17) with your hands on the mat directly under your shoulders and your knees directly under the hips. Your pelvis and spine should be neutral, and your hips should be flexed to 90 degrees. Pull your shoulders down and draw your belly button to your spine. Inhale in this position. **A**

2. While exhaling, use your abdominal muscles to curl the tailbone under and round (flex) the spine as you drop your head between your arms. **B**

3. Stay in this position and inhale, feeling the back muscles stretch.

4. Exhale once again, keeping the abdominal muscles engaged, and lift the tailbone and head to unroll the spine through neutral into a slightly arched (extended) position with your tailbone and head lifted slightly. **C**

5. Inhale again before repeating the movement.

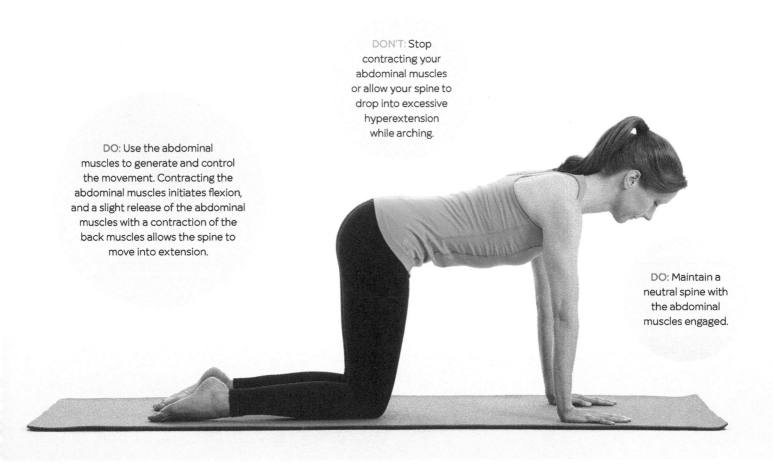

DON'T: Stop contracting your abdominal muscles or allow your spine to drop into excessive hyperextension while arching.

DO: Use the abdominal muscles to generate and control the movement. Contracting the abdominal muscles initiates flexion, and a slight release of the abdominal muscles with a contraction of the back muscles allows the spine to move into extension.

DO: Maintain a neutral spine with the abdominal muscles engaged.

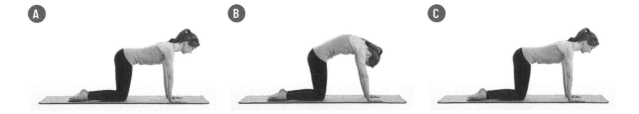

A   B   C

WATCHDOG (WARM-UP)

The Watchdog improves both core strength and balance. The spine and pelvis should remain stable while the opposite arm and leg lift off the ground. Be careful not to rotate one way or the other, arch your back, or curl your spine as the opposite arm and leg lift.

FOCUS: Maintain a neutral spine and keep your weight evenly balanced over the center of your mat.

REPETITIONS: 6 to 8

VISUALIZATION: Imagine your abdominal muscles tightening around your waist and spine like a corset. Then imagine this corset holding you still and stable as your arms and legs reach away. Imagine your spine getting longer.

PRECAUTIONS: If you have knee discomfort or injuries, you may need to kneel on cushions or a blanket, or perform this exercise standing with your hands on a chair.

1. Assume an all-fours position (page 17) with your hands on the mat directly under your shoulders and your knees directly under your hips. Your pelvis and spine should be neutral, and your hips should be flexed to 90 degrees. Pull your shoulders down and draw your belly button to your spine. Inhale in this position. **A**

2. While exhaling, lift your right arm straight in front of you and simultaneously lift your left leg off the ground in back of you, with your knee straight to create one long line between the fingertips of the right hand and the toes of the left foot. Maintain a neutral spine and keep your shoulders and hip bones facing the mat. **B**

3. Inhale as you return to the all-fours position. Check to make sure your pelvis and spine are neutral. **C**

4. Exhale as you lift your left arm straight out in front of you and extend your right leg straight back without changing the shape of your spine or rotating your powerhouse. **D**

5. Inhale as you return to the all-fours position. **E**

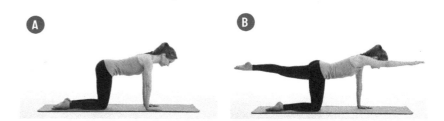

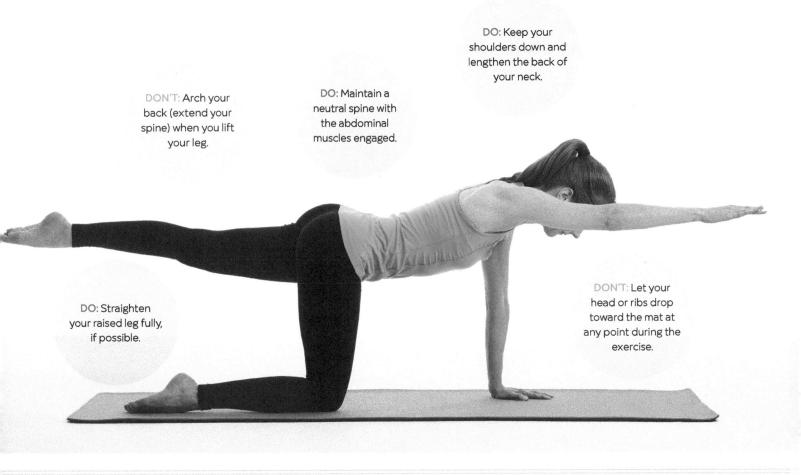

DON'T: Arch your back (extend your spine) when you lift your leg.

DO: Maintain a neutral spine with the abdominal muscles engaged.

DO: Keep your shoulders down and lengthen the back of your neck.

DO: Straighten your raised leg fully, if possible.

DON'T: Let your head or ribs drop toward the mat at any point during the exercise.

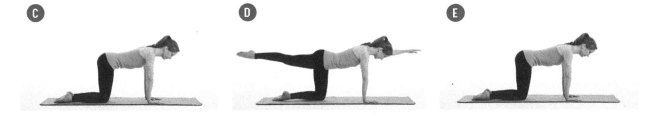

C

D

E

SHORT PLANK (WARM-UP)

The Short Plank targets both the abdominal muscles, to strengthen the core, and the muscles around the shoulders, to improve posture. When the abs are pulled in, the deepest layer of the abdominals is targeted. And when the shoulder blades (scapulas) are kept flat on the back, their bottom edges will not stick out, thus training your muscles for better posture.

FOCUS: Keep the shoulder joints and shoulder blades stable, the spine neutral, and the core engaged.

REPETITIONS: 3 to 5

VISUALIZATION: Imagine pressing the floor away without rounding your spine to engage the stabilizing muscles around the shoulder blades. Imagine your abdominal muscles drawing in toward your spine so strongly that you levitate and hover just above the ground.

PRECAUTIONS: If you have knee discomfort or injuries, you may need to kneel on cushions or a blanket.

1. Assume an all-fours position (page 17) with your hands on the mat directly under your shoulders and your knees directly under the hips. Flex your feet and tuck your toes. Your pelvis and spine should be neutral, and your hips should be flexed to 90 degrees. Pull your shoulders down and draw your belly button to your spine. Inhale in this position. **A**

2. As you exhale, press into your hands and feet to lift the knees just an inch off the floor. Maintain a neutral spine and keep your inner thighs activated. Imagine squeezing a Ping-Pong ball between your upper thighs. **B**

3. Lower your knees down to the mat, keeping the core engaged as you inhale. **C**

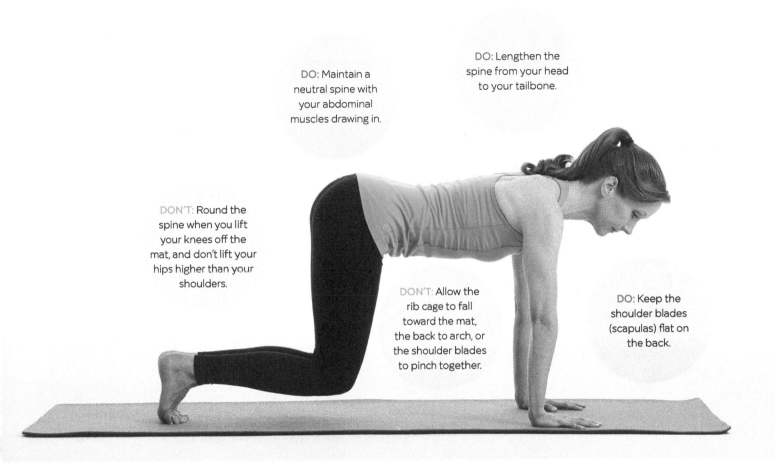

DO: Maintain a neutral spine with your abdominal muscles drawing in.

DO: Lengthen the spine from your head to your tailbone.

DON'T: Round the spine when you lift your knees off the mat, and don't lift your hips higher than your shoulders.

DON'T: Allow the rib cage to fall toward the mat, the back to arch, or the shoulder blades to pinch together.

DO: Keep the shoulder blades (scapulas) flat on the back.

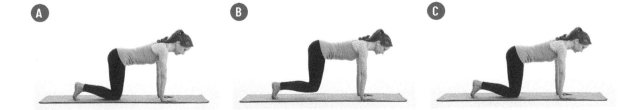

A B C

HALF SWAN (WARM-UP)

The Half Swan mobilizes the upper back (thoracic spine) into extension while stabilizing the lower back and pelvis. This combination of strengthening the muscles of the upper back and stabilizing the lower back and pelvis creates beautiful posture and relieves neck tension.

FOCUS: Lift just the head and shoulders off the mat, without the bottom rib lifting off the mat.

REPETITIONS: 4 to 6

VISUALIZATION: Imagine that your spine is getting longer as you lift your shoulders off the mat. Imagine reaching your heart forward to open the shoulders and chest.

PRECAUTIONS: Individuals with certain neck or back problems may find the start position uncomfortable. If you have neck problems, you can put a cushion under your head. If you experience lower-back discomfort, try putting a cushion under your hip bones.

1. Lie on your stomach with your legs together, or separated slightly if that's more comfortable. Place your hands just outside your shoulders and pull your belly button in toward your spine. Energize your legs but do not lift them. **A**

2. Inhale through your nose without changing anything from the start position. Just think of lengthening.

3. While exhaling, press into your hands and use the muscles of the upper back to lift your head and shoulders off the mat. Keep your chest open but your ribs closed. **B**

4. Inhale in this position, maintaining the pose.

5. Exhale and lower the head and shoulders down to the start position. **C**

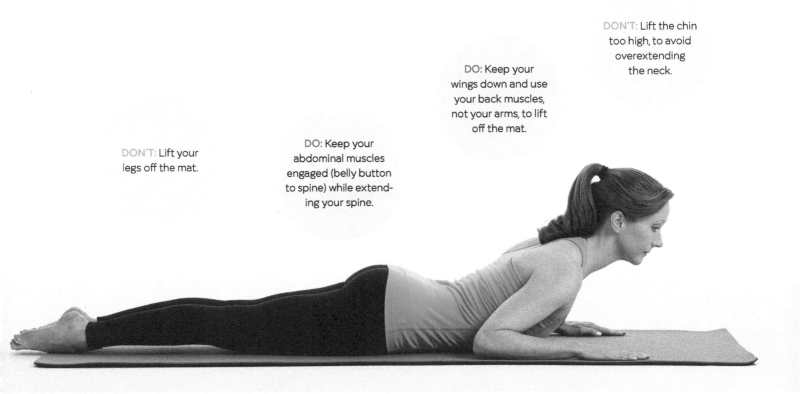

DON'T: Lift your legs off the mat.

DO: Keep your abdominal muscles engaged (belly button to spine) while extending your spine.

DO: Keep your wings down and use your back muscles, not your arms, to lift off the mat.

DON'T: Lift the chin too high, to avoid overextending the neck.

Ⓐ

Ⓑ

Ⓒ

HIP FLEXOR STRETCH (COOLDOWN)

Hip stretches relax and release the muscle groups that are active in stabilizing the pelvis in many Pilates exercises. When the muscles around the hip are tight, they can pull on the pelvis or the fascia in the lower back, contributing to lower-back pain or discomfort. This cooldown stretches these muscles to release any undue tension around the hips, creating a feeling of freedom in the both the hips and the lower back.

FOCUS: Release the muscles on the front of the hips after a hard workout.

REPETITIONS: 20 to 40 seconds, 3 to 4 times on each side

VISUALIZATION: Imagine that your muscle is a ball of yarn tied in a knot. With every exhale, envision the knot loosening slightly.

PRECAUTIONS: If you have had a hip replacement or a significant hip injury, consult with your doctor before doing this stretch.

1. Kneel on both knees, then step one foot forward to an upright kneeling position on one knee. The standing knee should be directly under the hip and both knees should form a right angle with the thigh bone. **A** If balance is difficult, use a chair for support. Otherwise, place both hands on your front knee. **B**

2. Breathing fluidly, ideally inhaling through your nose and exhaling through your mouth, gently lunge forward onto the front leg, keeping the torso as vertical as possible. You should feel a stretch in the front of the hip. **C**

3. Continuing to breathe smoothly, press into your front foot to come out of the stretch slightly, then move into the stretch again. Repeat this 3 to 4 times, using a chair for balance and support if necessary.

4. Repeat with the other leg.

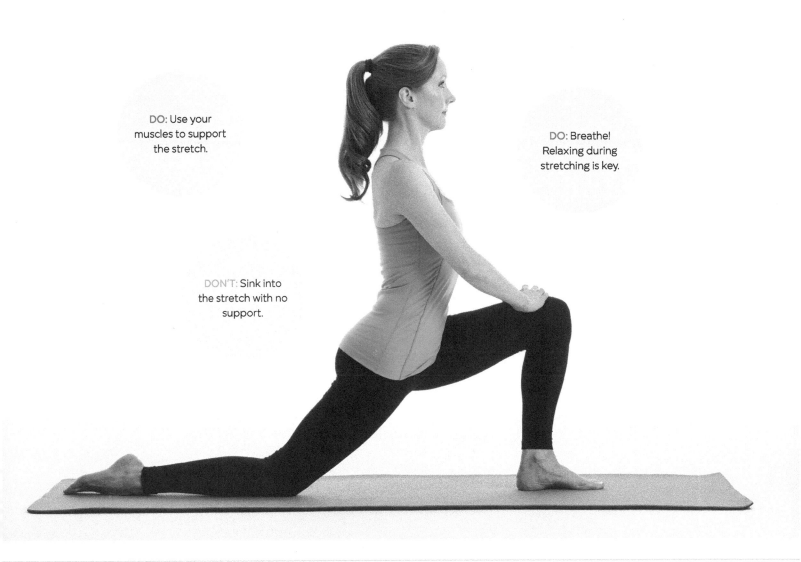

DO: Use your muscles to support the stretch.

DO: Breathe! Relaxing during stretching is key.

DON'T: Sink into the stretch with no support.

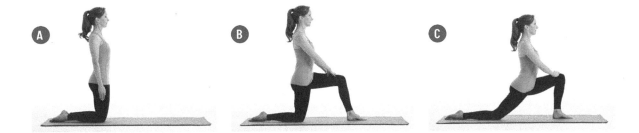

A

B

C

SIDE-HIP STRETCH (COOLDOWN)

While the previous hip stretch released the psoas and hip flexors at the front of the hip, these stretches for the sides of your hips release the tightness many feel in the gluteal (buttocks) muscles. These stretches also help release the fascia in the lower back, which can help alleviate lower back tension.

FOCUS: Release the muscles on the sides of the hips after a hard workout.

REPETITIONS: 20 to 40 seconds on each side

VISUALIZATION: Imagine that your muscle is a ball of yarn tied in a knot. With every exhale, envision the knot loosening slightly.

PRECAUTIONS: If you have had a hip replacement or a significant hip injury, consult with your doctor before doing this stretch.

1. Sit tall on the sit bones with the knees bent, feet flat on the mat in front of you. **A** Then stack one ankle on the opposite knee; the other ankle will be under your other knee. Your shins will be in line with your torso. **B**

2. Breathing fluidly, allow gravity to bring the top knee closer to the bottom ankle. Stay here for a few breaths, allowing your body to relax and your mind to center.

3. Bring the right ankle to the left and the left ankle to the right to stack the knees on top of one another in the center of the torso. **C**

4. Breathe smoothly, aiming to get both sit bones to the floor gently, without forcing. Remain in the stretch for a few breaths, relaxing. (Optional: Lean forward to intensify the stretch.)

5. Repeat both stretches with the other leg on top.

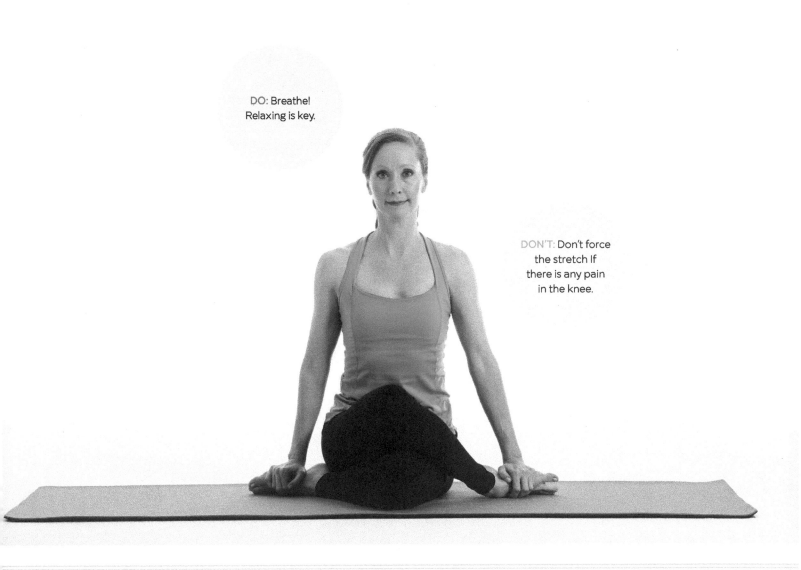

DO: Breathe! Relaxing is key.

DON'T: Don't force the stretch If there is any pain in the knee.

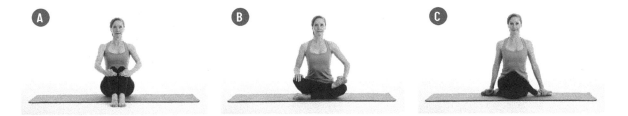

A   B   C

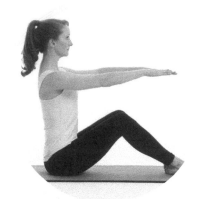

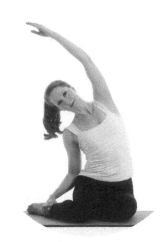

CHAPTER

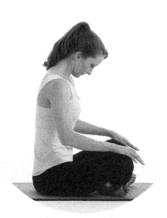

INTRODUCTORY PROGRAM

THIS PROGRAM BUILDS A STRONG FOUNDATION for your Pilates practice, with exercises that focus on deep core strengthening and proper technique. Most of the exercises are modified versions of their Level 1 or Level 2 counterparts to help build strength and awareness without increasing difficulty too soon. Expect some exercises to be easier for you than others. This is completely normal, as we all have different bodies and different genetic makeups that cause us to move more comfortably in some ways than in others. With this in mind, we've included exercises that mobilize the spine in all directions while building strength within the full range of motion. Once you are able to perform the introductory exercises with proper form and ease, you will be ready to move to Level 1.

INTRODUCTORY PROGRAM SEQUENCE

This Introductory Sequence teaches the fundamentals of Pilates principles with careful attention to placement of the body in all exercises. It will ensure you build a solid foundation to help you reap all the benefits Pilates has to offer. As you look at the sequence layout, you will notice that it introduces all spinal movements: bending forward, backward, side bending and rotating. You will begin to learn how your powerhouse supports you in all movements you encounter in life.

If you find certain elements of the Pilates technique difficult to achieve, that's okay! Be patient with yourself. Take note of what you find challenging and take the time to do the exercises correctly. At this level, do not worry about transitions. It is more important to get the technique into your body. The transitions will flow naturally after that.

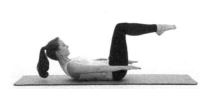
THE HUNDRED, MODIFIED,
page 50

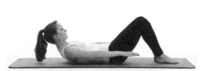
THE ROLL-UP, MODIFIED
page 52

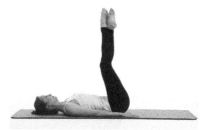
THE ROLLOVER, MODIFIED
page 54

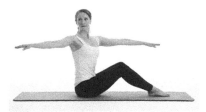

SPINE TWIST, MODIFIED
page 56

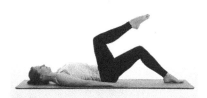

SINGLE-LEG CIRCLES, MODIFIED
page 58

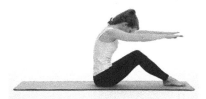

ROLLING LIKE A BALL, MODIFIED
page 60

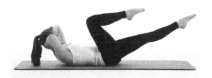

SINGLE-LEG STRETCH, MODIFIED
page 62

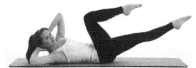

CRISS-CROSS, MODIFIED
page 64

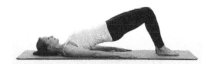

SHOULDER BRIDGE, MODIFIED
page 66

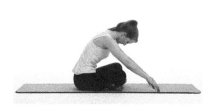

SPINE STRETCH FORWARD,
MODIFIED
page 68

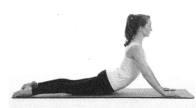

SWAN DIVE, MODIFIED
page 70

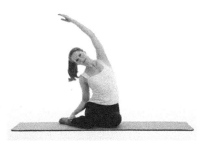

MERMAID STRETCH
page 72

THE HUNDRED, MODIFIED

In the full version of the Hundred (page 80), the legs are completely straight, but at this level, the legs remain bent to reduce the burden on your abdominal muscles. The legs are heavier when straight; keeping them bent allows you to focus on keeping your abdominal muscles pulled in as flat as possible.

FOCUS: Keep your abdominal muscles engaged and pulled flat to your spine, and keep your shoulders down and tension out of your neck for the full 100 count.

REPETITIONS: 10 sets of 5 inhales and 5 exhales, up to the count of 100

VISUALIZATION: Imagine your arms bouncing on a small ball placed under the top of your arms. Imagine your abs getting flatter and flatter as you progress.

PRECAUTIONS: Avoid this exercise if you have been advised by a doctor not to lift your head off the mat. Also, if you have been told by a medical professional not to flex your spine, you should skip this one.

1. Lie on your back with your knees bent and feet flat on the floor, sit-bones distance apart. Keep your pelvis neutral. Engage your abdominal muscles, flattening them, and draw your hip bones closer to your ribs to achieve the imprint position. Your arms should be by your sides. **A**

2. Lift one leg, then the other, up into tabletop position, so your hips and knees are bent at 90 degrees with your shins parallel to the floor. Do not allow your hip bones to fall away from your ribs. **B**

3. As you inhale, tuck your chin to chest, lengthening the back of your neck.

4. While exhaling, use the abdominal muscles to lift the head and shoulders off the mat, simultaneously lifting the arms to shoulder height and maintaining the strong connection between the ribs and hips. **C**

5. Take 5 short "sips" of air in through the nose for 5 counts, pumping your arms up and down slightly.

6. Then, continuing the pumping motion of the arms, exhale through the mouth for 5 counts, blowing out a little bit of air each time. Continue for 9 more sets.

7. After your last set, inhale deeply to curl the head and shoulders off the mat even more.

8. As you exhale, lower the head and shoulders down to the mat. Return one leg, then the other, to the mat. **D**

A

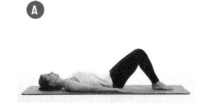

DON'T: Let the ribs pop out, allow the hip bones to fall away from the ribs, or allow the lower back to arch (extend).

DO: Feel the energy all the way through the tips of your fingers and toes.

DO: Maintain a strong abdominal connection throughout.

STOP: If it gets too hard to continue.

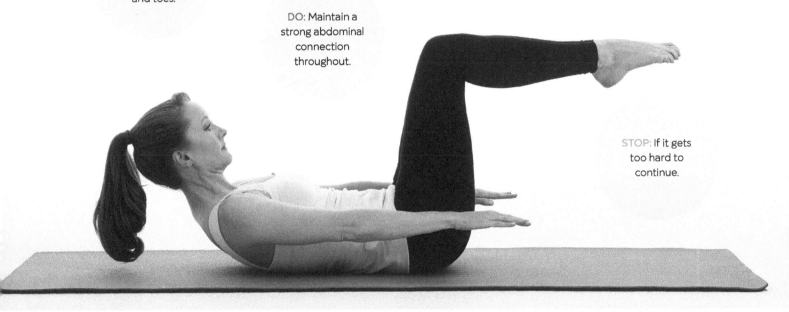

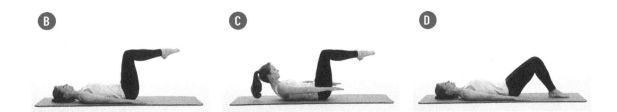

THE ROLL-UP, MODIFIED

The Roll-Up consists of two distinct skills: rolling UP from lying on your back and rolling DOWN from a seated position. The full Roll-Up is in Level 1 (page 82). We have modified the Roll-Up in the Introductory Program to roll just the head and shoulders off the mat. By focusing on a half roll-up, you'll build strength while maintaining the proper form of keeping your belly button to your spine and wings down. Once you master successful execution of this modified version, you will be prepared to take on the challenge of the full Roll-Up.

FOCUS: Create a smooth, even curve of the spine while maintaining flat abs and fluid breath.

REPETITIONS: 4 to 6

VISUALIZATION: Imagine your spine is a string of pearls that lifts off a dresser one pearl at a time and is placed back down one pearl at a time.

PRECAUTIONS: Individuals with neck injuries may want to skip this and jump to Rolling Like a Ball, Modified (page 60) to avoid strain on the neck. If you've been advised to avoid rotation due to lower back or disc injuries, skip this exercise until you are cleared by a medical professional. Always work in a pain-free range of motion.

1. Begin lying on your back with your legs together, knees bent, and feet flat on the floor. The pelvis and spine are neutral. **A**

2. As you inhale, tuck the chin slightly and pull in the abdominal muscles like a corset.

3. As you exhale, lift the head and shoulders off the mat while keeping the pelvis neutral. **B**

4. Inhale to maintain that position.

5. Exhale to lower the head and shoulders back down to the mat with control. **C**

DON'T: "Hinge" the head and shoulders off the mat— maintain the curve of the spine.

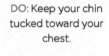

DO: Keep your chin tucked toward your chest.

DO: Keep your belly button pulled in to your spine.

DON'T: Let your abdominal muscles pop.

DO: Focus on a smooth, even curve of the spine.

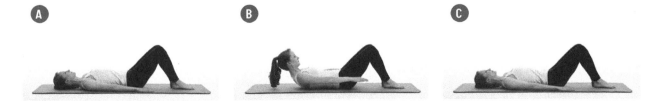

A

B

C

THE ROLLOVER, MODIFIED

This move strengthens the muscles of the lower abdomen to prepare for the full Rollover, which can be found in Level 2 (page 118). The Rollover is a challenging exercise designed to strengthen the lower abs and core and develop control as well as flexibility of the spine. This modified version will help you build the powerhouse strength needed to perform the full Rollover precisely and without injury.

FOCUS: Maintain flat abs and core control as your hips lift and lower. Focus on performing the movement slowly and deliberately, using the abdominal muscles to lift the hips.

REPETITIONS: 6 to 8

VISUALIZATION: Imagine your toes being pulled straight toward the ceiling.

PRECAUTIONS: If you have lower-back problems, start with the hips elevated slightly or skip this exercise altogether.

1. Lie on your back with your legs bent, feet flat on the floor, and arms by your sides. Inhale as you feel length in your spine, then exhale and engage the abdominal muscles to flatten the back to the mat and roll the hip bones up toward the ribs. **A**

2. Inhale as you lift one leg up into tabletop position, and then exhale to bring the other leg up into tabletop position. **B**

3. Inhale and exhale and straighten your knees slightly, then cross your right ankle over the left, reaching your legs toward the ceiling. **C**

4. Inhale to pull your belly button to your spine to fortify the abdominal connection.

5. As you exhale, use your abdominal muscles to contract the abs and lift your hips off the mat, reaching your toes to the ceiling while keeping your legs slightly bent. **D**

6. Inhale as you return your hips to the mat.

7. After 3 to 4 repetitions, switch your feet and repeat. **E**

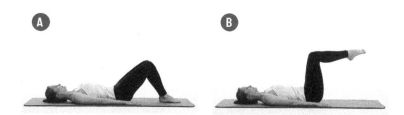

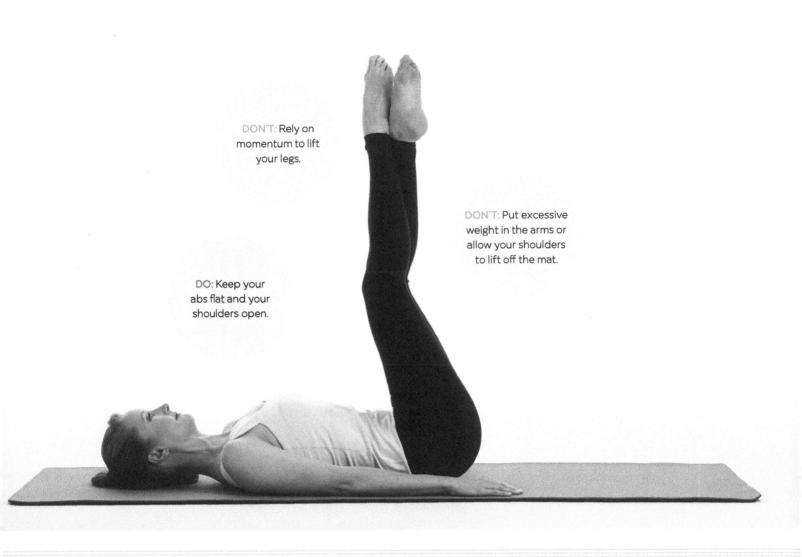

DON'T: Rely on momentum to lift your legs.

DON'T: Put excessive weight in the arms or allow your shoulders to lift off the mat.

DO: Keep your abs flat and your shoulders open.

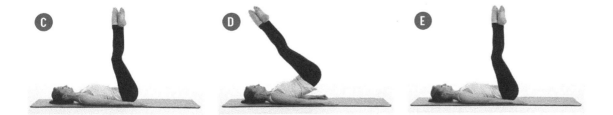

C D E

SPINE TWIST, MODIFIED

The Spine Twist (page 96) teaches pure rotation of the spine by the controlled action of the abdominal muscles. It also trains the deep muscles of the abdomen and spine to support the body in proper posture and alignment. In this modified version, the exercise is performed in a seated position to eliminate any discomfort in the hips or legs.

FOCUS: Isolate the rotation of the spine above the pelvis without popping the ribs (extending the spine) or bending to the side.

REPETITIONS: 4 to 6 in each direction

VISUALIZATION: Imagine the space between each vertebra increasing throughout the movement. Visualize growing taller or spiraling upward throughout the exercise.

PRECAUTIONS: If you've been advised to avoid rotation due to lower-back or disc injuries, skip this exercise until cleared by a medical professional. Always work in a pain-free range of motion.

1. Sit on top of the sit bones, either with your knees bent and feet flat on the floor, or up on cushions so that the pelvis and spine remain neutral, with your legs out as straight as possible. Ideally, the legs should be squeezing together, but in case of discomfort, separate the legs slightly. **A**

2. Reach your arms straight out to the sides where your fingers can still be seen in your peripheral vision. Pull in your abdominal muscles, slide your shoulders down your back (wings down), and sit as tall as possible, lengthening through the top of your head. **B**

3. Inhale 3 times in succession, like you're taking 3 sniffs of air through your nose to fill the lungs. (This is similar to the breath in the Hundred, Modified, page 50.) While inhaling, twist your spine to the left without allowing your hips to shift. At the end range of rotation, inhale with 2 more sniffs and gently increase your range of rotation. Turn your head to the left as well, looking toward your left fingers. **C**

4. Exhale smoothly, rotating the spine in the opposite direction to return to the start position. Make sure that your wings are down and your abdominal muscles are flat. **D**

5. Repeat the movement to the right, **E** inhaling 3 times while rotating to the right and exhaling to return to the start position. **F**

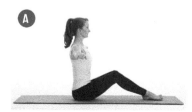
A

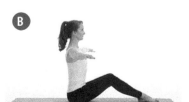
B

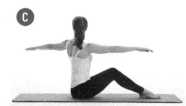
C

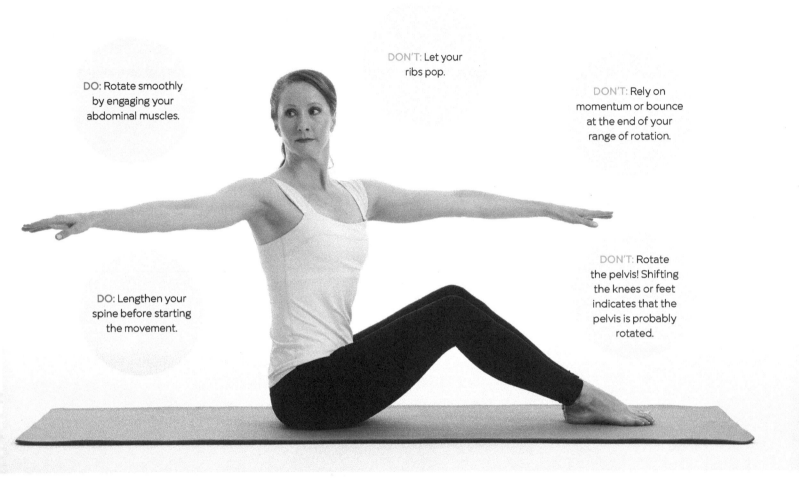

DO: Rotate smoothly by engaging your abdominal muscles.

DON'T: Let your ribs pop.

DON'T: Rely on momentum or bounce at the end of your range of rotation.

DO: Lengthen your spine before starting the movement.

DON'T: Rotate the pelvis! Shifting the knees or feet indicates that the pelvis is probably rotated.

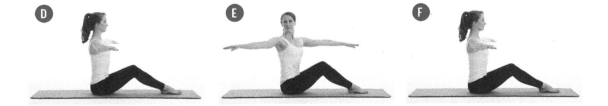

D   E   F

SINGLE-LEG CIRCLES, MODIFIED

Single-Leg Circles, a Level 1 exercise (page 84), challenges the stability of the torso against the movement of the leg while providing support for the lower back. This exercise is great for improving balance. In the modified version, the knee is bent to make the weight of the leg lighter on the abdominal muscles. This allows you to focus on stability over range of motion. The circles should be kept small initially so you can slowly gain strength and stability.

FOCUS: Keep the pelvis and spine neutral and stable against the circular movement of the leg.

REPETITIONS: 4 to 6 in each direction, on both sides

VISUALIZATION: To maintain stability of the neutral pelvis, imagine that your pelvis and tailbone are very heavy and immovable. Imagine that a pencil is attached to your femur drawing small circles on the ceiling.

PRECAUTIONS: If you experience instability in the lumbar spine, perform the exercise in the imprint position.

1. Lie on your back on the mat with your legs sit-bones distance apart, both knees bent and feet flat on the floor, and your arms by your sides. Your pelvis and spine should be neutral, and your abdominal muscles should be pulled in tight. **A**

2. Exhale and lift your right leg into the air, keeping the knee bent. Your femur should form right angles with your body and your shin. **B**

3. While inhaling smoothly, bring the right knee slightly toward your body, then across the midline of your body and down slightly, as if you're drawing a semicircle on the ceiling. **C**

4. While exhaling smoothly, complete the other half of the circle by moving the femur away from your midline and back up to the top of the circle. **D**

5. Continue in this direction, inhaling for the first half of the circle and exhaling for the second half of the circle, for 4 to 6 repetitions. Then reverse the direction of the circles, inhaling when the femur moves away from your midline and exhaling when it moves up toward the midline. Continue in this direction for 4 to 6 repetitions.

6. Repeat with the opposite leg.

A

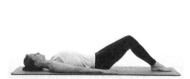

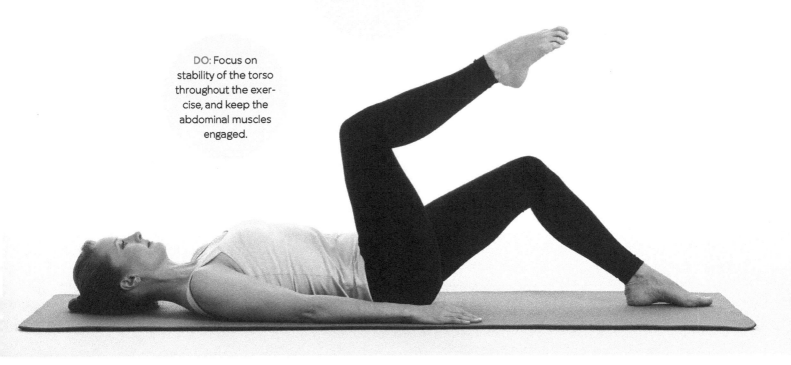

DON'T: Sacrifice stability for increased range of motion.

DO: Focus on stability of the torso throughout the exercise, and keep the abdominal muscles engaged.

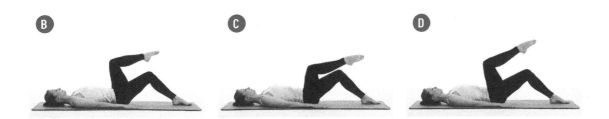

B

C

D

ROLLING LIKE A BALL, MODIFIED

This modified exercise teaches the proper muscular engagement necessary for performing the full Rolling Like a Ball exercise (page 86) correctly with maximal control and minimal momentum. It strengthens and tones the abdominal muscles while increasing spinal flexibility.

FOCUS: Keep abdominal control throughout the range of motion.

REPETITIONS: 4 to 6

VISUALIZATION: Anatomically speaking, "upper abs" and "lower abs" are not technically muscles! However, for visualization purposes, imagine contracting the lower abs more when rolling back and contracting the upper abs more when returning. Picture the abdominal muscles as both the accelerators and the brakes!

PRECAUTIONS: If you've been advised to avoid rotation due to lower-back or disc injuries, skip this exercise until cleared by a medical professional. Always work in a pain-free range of motion.

1. Sit tall with your weight even on both sit bones. Keep your pelvis neutral and your knees bent with your feet flat on the mat. Ideally, your legs are squeezing together, but if you feel discomfort, separate your legs slightly. Reach your arms in front of your body and sit as tall as possible with your wings down. **A**

2. While keeping the pelvis neutral (i.e., staying on top of the sit bones without rolling backward), pull your abdominal muscles in. Scoop in the abs and curl the spine over the knees, creating a C-curve of the spine. This is the start position, and you will keep this C-curve for the duration of the exercises. **B**

3. While exhaling, contract the abdominal muscles, maintain the C-curve of the spine, and roll backward off your sit bones, feeling your weight move to your tailbone and then your sacrum. Continue to roll back as far as you can (without falling backward onto the mat), maintaining the C-curve and keeping your feet on the mat. **C**

4. Inhale at the end range to hold the position, keeping the C-curve of the spine and keeping the abdominal muscles engaged and flat.

5. Then exhale and increase the contraction in the abdominals to bring the weight of the body back to the sit bones, maintaining the C-curve of the spine throughout the motion. You will be looking at your knees. **D** Repeat.

6. To finish, roll up, one vertebra at a time, until the spine is neutral.

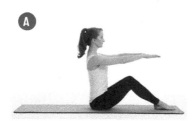

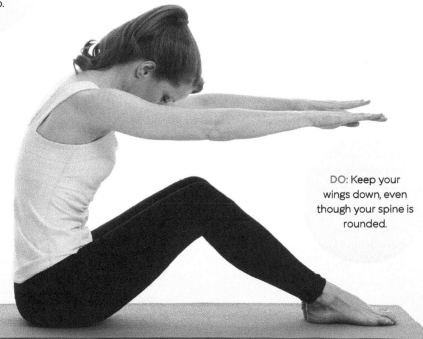

DO: Control the range of motion using the strength of your abdominal muscles.

DO: Keep the abdominal muscles drawn in and up without letting them pop.

DON'T: Lose the C-curve or overly round the shoulders.

DO: Keep your wings down, even though your spine is rounded.

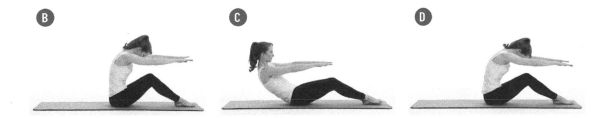

B

C

D

SINGLE-LEG STRETCH, MODIFIED

The Single-Leg Stretch (page 88) builds abdominal strength, tones the legs, and challenges the stability of the spine. The key to toning your legs is straightening them fully in each repetition. In this modified version, the pace is slower, and you'll support your head with your hands to avoid strain in the neck while you strengthen your abdominal muscles.

FOCUS: Maintain a strong imprint position against the weight of your extended leg.

REPETITIONS: 8 to 10

VISUALIZATION: Imagine the end points of a line, between the knee coming toward the chest and the foot of the extended leg, reaching away from each other. Imagine curling up higher with each repetition.

PRECAUTIONS: If you've been advised to avoid rotation due to lower-back or disc injuries, skip this exercise until you are cleared by a medical professional. Always work in a pain-free range of motion.

1. Lie on your back on the mat with your legs sit-bones distance apart, both knees bent and feet flat on the floor, and arms by your sides. **A** Move to the imprint position. Inhale and lift one leg up into tabletop position, then exhale and lift the other leg up into tabletop. **B** Your femurs should form right angles with your body and your shins. Place both hands behind your head with your thumbs at your hairline and elbows reaching wide. Lift your head and shoulders off the mat to assume the start position. **C**

2. While exhaling, extend your right leg straight out into a low diagonal and draw the left knee closer to your forehead, simultaneously curling up higher off the mat. Lower the right leg only as far as you can simultaneously maintain stability in the low back. **D**

3. Inhale and return both legs to the start position, being careful not to let your head and shoulders drop. **E**

4. Exhale and extend the left leg out into a low diagonal, and curl up higher while bringing the right knee closer to your forehead. **F**

5. Inhale and return both legs to the start position, being careful not to let your head and shoulders drop. **G** Repeat.

6. After you finish your repetitions, lower your head and shoulders to the mat, then lower your legs, one at a time.

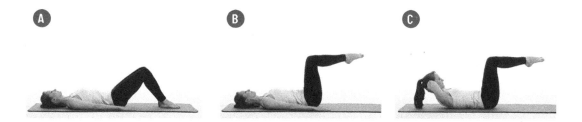

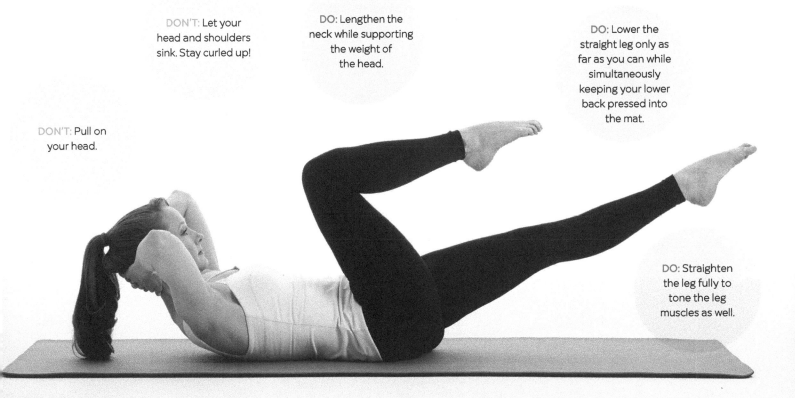

DON'T: Let your head and shoulders sink. Stay curled up!

DON'T: Pull on your head.

DO: Lengthen the neck while supporting the weight of the head.

DO: Lower the straight leg only as far as you can while simultaneously keeping your lower back pressed into the mat.

DO: Straighten the leg fully to tone the leg muscles as well.

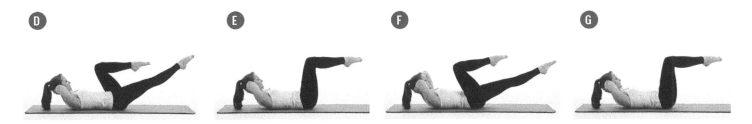

D **E** **F** **G**

CRISS-CROSS, MODIFIED

The Criss-Cross (page 90) builds on the skills developed in the Single-Leg Stretch (page 88). This modified version similarly builds on the foundation learned in the Single-Leg Stretch, Modified (page 62). The obliques are targeted more, spinal flexibility is increased, and the legs are further toned.

FOCUS: Maintain a strong imprint against the weight of one extended leg while increasing the rotation of the spine.

REPETITIONS: 8 to 10

VISUALIZATION: Imagine the end points of a line, between the knee coming toward the chest and the foot of the extended leg, reaching away from each other. Imagine curling up higher with each repetition.

PRECAUTIONS: If you've been advised to avoid rotation due to lower-back or disc injuries, skip this exercise until you are cleared by a medical professional. Always work in a pain-free range of motion.

1. Lie on your back on the mat with your legs sit-bones distance apart, both knees bent and feet flat on the floor, and arms by your sides. **A** Move to the imprint position. Inhale and lift one leg up into tabletop position, then exhale and lift the other leg up into tabletop. Your femurs should form right angles with your body and your shins. **B** Place both hands behind your head with your thumbs at your hairline and elbows reaching wide. Lift your head and shoulders off the mat to assume the start position. **C**

2. While exhaling, extend the right leg straight out on a low diagonal and draw the left knee closer to your chest, simultaneously twisting your shoulders and rib cage toward the left knee. Focus on the right shoulder reaching toward the left knee. **D**

3. Inhale and return to the start position, being careful not to let your head and shoulders drop. **E**

4. Then exhale and extend the left leg straight out on a low diagonal and bring your right knee closer to your twist while twisting to the right, aiming the left shoulder toward the right knee. **F**

5. Inhale and return both legs to the start position. **G** Repeat.

6. After you finish your repetitions, lower your head and shoulders to the mat, then lower the legs one at a time.

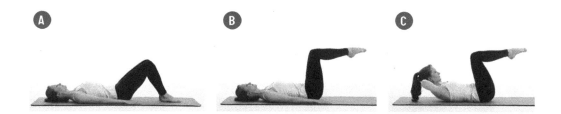

A **B** **C**

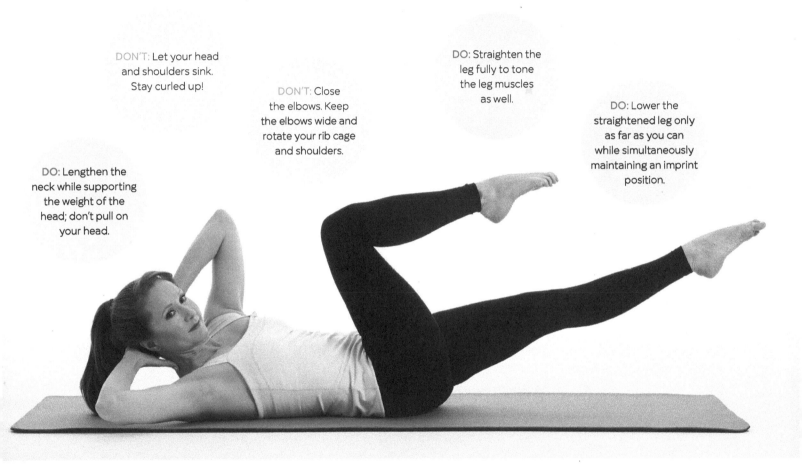

DON'T: Let your head and shoulders sink. Stay curled up!

DON'T: Close the elbows. Keep the elbows wide and rotate your rib cage and shoulders.

DO: Straighten the leg fully to tone the leg muscles as well.

DO: Lower the straightened leg only as far as you can while simultaneously maintaining an imprint position.

DO: Lengthen the neck while supporting the weight of the head; don't pull on your head.

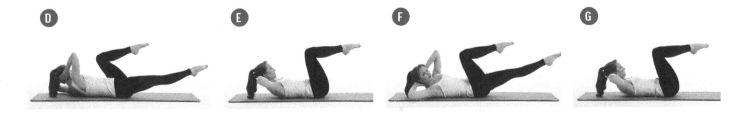

D   E   F   G

SHOULDER BRIDGE, MODIFIED

Planks are a staple of any core-strengthening routine, and the modified Shoulder Bridge is an excellent way to start planking to build strength in the glutes, in the hamstrings to lift the hips, and in the core to maintain the lower spine and pelvis in neutral throughout the movement.

FOCUS: Create a straight line between your armpits and your knees and hold that position with ease.

REPETITIONS: 4 to 6

VISUALIZATION: Imagine you are being lifted from two hooks, one on each hip bone; as the hips lower, imagine folding at the hips like a rag doll.

PRECAUTIONS: If you have knee problems or extremely tight quads, you may feel discomfort in your knees during this exercise. If this is the case, work in a pain-free range of motion by placing your feet farther away from the hips.

1. Lie on your back with your knees bent and feet flat on the floor sit-bones distance apart, and arms by your side. Your pelvis and spine should be neutral, with your head and neck relaxed. **A**

2. Inhale, pull in your abs, and lengthen your spine.

3. As you exhale, keep your spine neutral (i.e., don't roll up!), press into your feet, and contract your glutes to lift your hips up toward the ceiling, ultimately creating a straight line from your armpits to your knees. **B**

4. While maintaining this position, inhale to feel length from the shoulders to the knees and through the spine and hip joint.

5. Exhale and slowly lower the hips to the mat, maintaining a neutral spine throughout. **C**

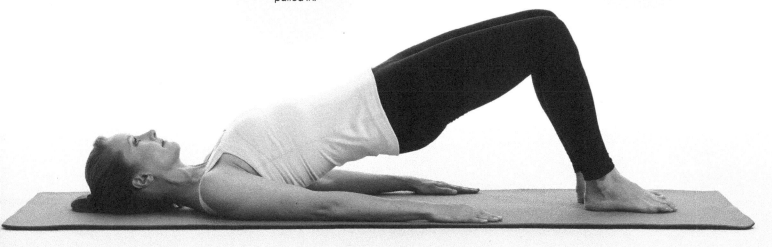

DO: Maintain a neutral pelvis and spine throughout the movement; don't roll up or down.

DO: Keep your abdominal muscles pulled in.

DON'T: Lift your hips so high that the lumbar spine arches (moves into extension).

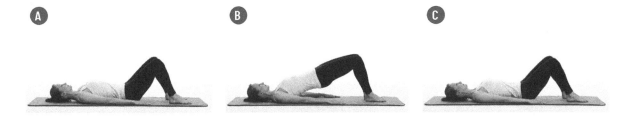

A

B

C

SPINE STRETCH FORWARD, MODIFIED

The Spine Stretch Forward is a Level 1 exercise (page 98) that builds awareness of the muscles on the front and back of the spine. It helps cultivate both a flexible spine and improved posture over time. In the introductory, modified version, we've altered the start position to help achieve a neutral pelvis and to eliminate any discomfort in the hips, hamstrings, or lower back.

FOCUS: Roll down and then up through the spine, one vertebra at a time.

REPETITIONS: 4 to 6

VISUALIZATION: Imagine that your spine is a piece of tape on a wall— you peel it off the wall slowly, and then press it back to the wall from the bottom up.

PRECAUTIONS: If you've been diagnosed with a spinal condition, osteoporosis, any disc herniation, or have an exaggerated kyphosis of the thoracic spine, skip this exercise.

1. Sit either in a chair or cross-legged on a cushion—whichever seated position allows the exercise to begin with your pelvis and spine in a neutral position. Rest your hands comfortably on your thighs, with your legs parallel and slightly wider than hip distance apart. **A**

2. Inhale and pull your belly button to your spine, lengthening through the top of your head.

3. Exhale as you roll down one vertebra at a time, starting by nodding the chin toward the chest and then rounding through the upper back, **B** mid back, **C** and lower back. Keep the pelvis neutral. **D**

4. Inhale in this position, maintaining the abdominal connection and the shape of the spine, while feeling the breath fill the back and sides of the ribs.

5. Exhale to "unroll" the torso back to vertical, rolling up one vertebra at a time. **E**

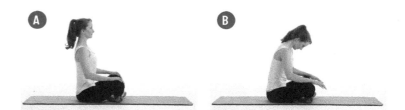

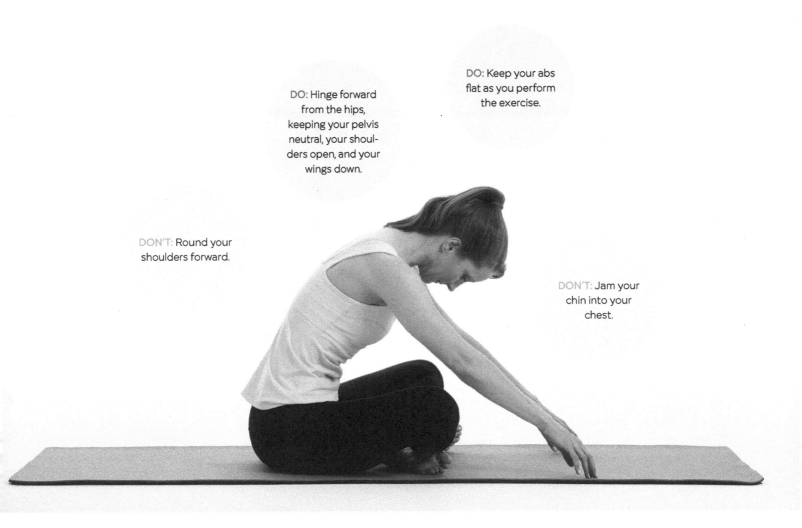

DO: Hinge forward from the hips, keeping your pelvis neutral, your shoulders open, and your wings down.

DO: Keep your abs flat as you perform the exercise.

DON'T: Round your shoulders forward.

DON'T: Jam your chin into your chest.

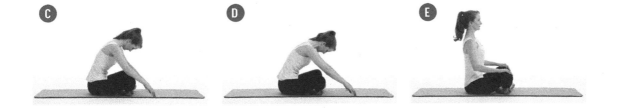

C

D

E

SWAN DIVE, MODIFIED

The Swan Dive is an advanced exercise that challenges spinal flexibility, core strength, and body awareness. Both this exercise and the Swan Dive 2, Modified in Level 2 (page 122) are building blocks for Joseph Pilates's advanced classical Swan Dive. In this modified version, spinal flexibility is the focus. The exercise opens the front line of the body, countering the effects of sitting all day. It also strengthens the muscles of the back and tones the glutes and hamstrings (delivering a bit of a butt lift!).

FOCUS: Move the spine into its own full, even extension with no pain or discomfort.

REPETITIONS: 4 to 6

VISUALIZATION: Imagine that you are getting longer, lengthening through the top of your head as you move the spine into extension.

PRECAUTIONS: Individuals with exaggerated kyphosis of the thoracic spine may need to modify this exercise. Individuals with exaggerated lordosis of the lumbar spine may need to reduce the range of motion or skip the exercise. If you've been advised against extension of the spine (back bending), be sure to limit the range of motion and support the position with your abdominal muscles.

1. Lie on your stomach with your legs shoulder-width apart and your knees pointing out to the sides. Your pelvis and spine should be neutral. Place your hands on the floor just outside the shoulders with your elbows bent. **Ⓐ**

2. Inhale to pull your belly button to your spine, and lengthen through the top of your head.

3. As you exhale, press into your hands to lift your head, shoulders, and as much of your rib cage and possibly hip bones off the mat, as your flexibility allows. Your elbows may or may not straighten fully. **Ⓑ**

4. Inhale at your end range.

5. Exhale to bend the elbows and lower your torso back down to the start position. **Ⓒ**

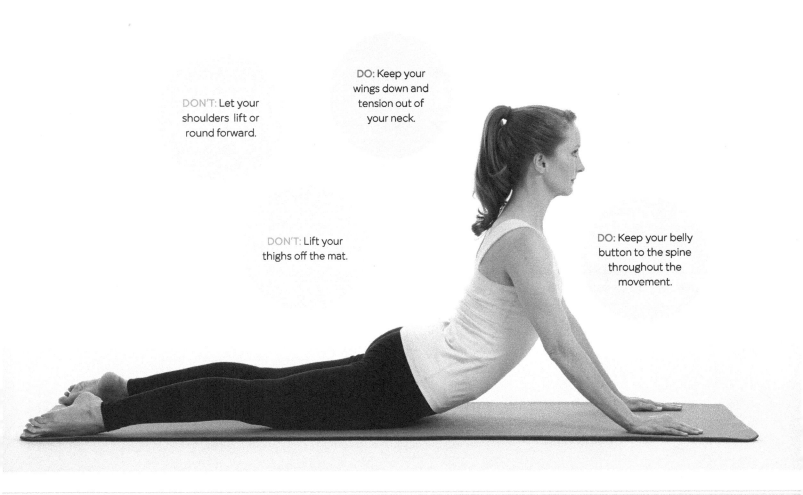

DON'T: Let your shoulders lift or round forward.

DO: Keep your wings down and tension out of your neck.

DON'T: Lift your thighs off the mat.

DO: Keep your belly button to the spine throughout the movement.

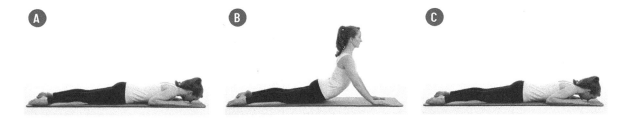

A

B

C

MERMAID STRETCH

This stretch increases the flexibility of the spine in side bending, and increases the space between your ribs to bring a feeling of expansive breath.

FOCUS: Increase your range of motion by side bending the spine without bending forward or rotating.

REPETITIONS: 3 to 5 on each side

VISUALIZATION: Picture how a geyser or a water fountain shoots up before arching over; envision this while side bending.

PRECAUTIONS: If you've been advised to avoid side bending due to spinal issues (herniated discs, injury, etc.), then work only in a pain-free range of motion or skip the exercise.

1. Sit on top of your sit bones with your knees bent and feet flat on the floor, pelvis and spine neutral. **A** Keeping the spine neutral (although the pelvis will shift), swing your legs to the right to bring the heels of both feet to the outside of your right hip. Your left heel will be closest to the right hip, with the right heel just outside of the left foot. Keep your weight mainly on the left hip; however, try to reach the right sit bone to the floor. Make sure your spine is as straight as possible, the abdominal muscles are pulled in and up, and your wings are down. Place your right hand on your right ankle and lift your left arm overhead. This is the start position for performing the mermaid stretch to the right. **B** (Reverse these directions for the left side.)

2. Take a deep inhale, then reach up farther through the left arm and lengthen your spine. **C**

3. While exhaling smoothly, engage your abdominal muscles and side bend to the right, keeping your left arm by your left ear and reaching your fingertips toward the opposite wall. **D**

4. Inhale deeply and stay in the stretch, reaching farther and expanding the ribs on the left side.

5. Exhale fully and return to the start position. **E**

6. Swing the legs around to repeat on the other side.

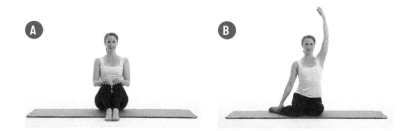

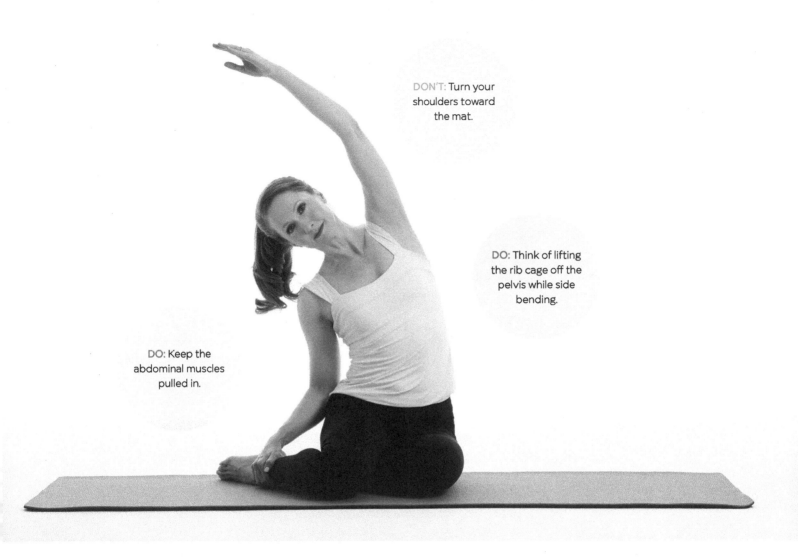

DON'T: Turn your shoulders toward the mat.

DO: Think of lifting the rib cage off the pelvis while side bending.

DO: Keep the abdominal muscles pulled in.

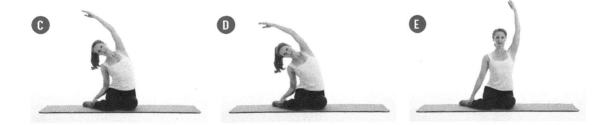

C

D

E

ASSESSING YOUR PROGRESS

Just as the foundation of a building takes months to build while the rest of the build-ing seems to spring up very quickly, so too does the foundation of Pilates take time to establish. We've created this questionnaire to inspire you, not discourage you! It is just as much about awareness as it is about skill development. Every *body* is different. It's more important to understand the concepts of Pilates than to perform every exercise "perfectly."

If you answer "yes" to all of the questions below, congratulations—it's time to move to Level 1! If you answer "yes" to most but not all of the questions, go ahead and move to Level 1, but stick with the Introductory Program exercises for anything you answered "no" to. If most of your answers are "no", don't fret! Just stick with the Introductory Program for one more week to make sure your core is strong enough to move to the next level.

No matter how your self-assessment looks, remember you're making important progress.

1. Does the concept of imprint make sense to you? Can you maintain an imprint position in exercises like the Hundred, Modified (page 50) or Criss-Cross, Modified (page 64)?

2. Can you keep your abs engaged and flat in all repetitions of the exercises without allowing them to pop? Are you aware when they do pop?

3. Does the term "wings down" make sense? Do you have an awareness of the muscles that make this happen?

4. Do you know how and when to modify for yourself? Are you aware of your thresholds? For instance, when to stop lowering the legs to protect your lower back? When to limit range of motion in rotation, back bending, and side bending?

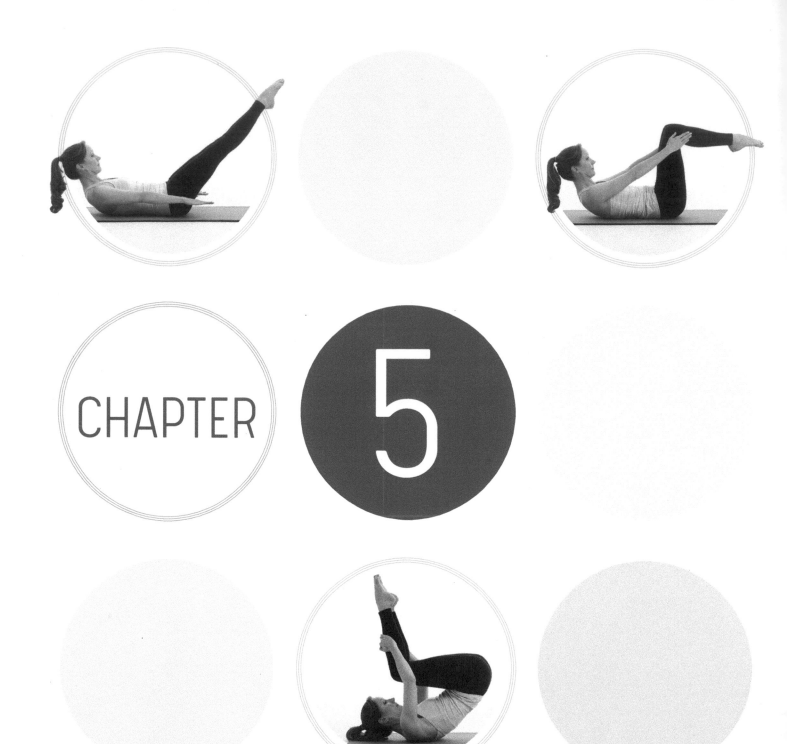

CHAPTER

5

LEVEL 1 PROGRAM

THE LEVEL 1 PROGRAM BUILDS UPON the technique and strength learned in the Introductory Program to help you achieve flatter abs, increased muscle tone throughout the body, and enhanced flexibility. Expect the exercises to be more challenging, both in terms of strength demands and body awareness. Best of all, expect to start feeling like a true Pilates enthusiast!

LEVEL 1 SEQUENCE

While the Introductory Sequence lays a solid foundation, the Level 1 sequence safely intensifies these exercises and introduces new exercises to deepen your understanding of Pilates principles and further strengthen your core. You may have noticed that as you progressed with the Introductory Sequence, the time it took you to complete all of the exercises decreased! This shows that your body has "downloaded" the technique, and you actually can move through the exercises smoothly without losing good form.

With the exception of Shoulder Bridge, Modified, and Mermaid Stretch, all exercises in the Level 1 sequence are more challenging versions of their Introductory Sequence counterparts. While practicing the Level 1 sequence, be mindful of moving from one exercise to the next with intent: Keep your core engaged, your breath smooth and flowing, and your movements deliberate.

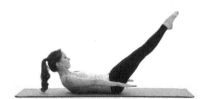

THE HUNDRED
page 80

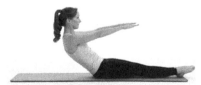

THE ROLL-UP
page 82

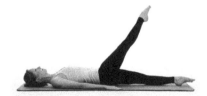

SINGLE-LEG CIRCLES
page 84

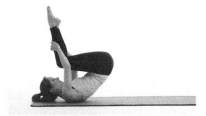

ROLLING LIKE A BALL
page 86

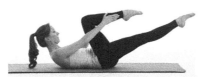

SINGLE-LEG STRETCH
page 88

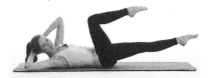

CRISS-CROSS
page 90

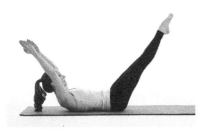

DOUBLE-LEG STRETCH, MODIFIED
page 92

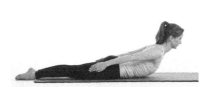

BREAST STROKE
page 94

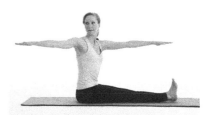

SPINE TWIST
page 96

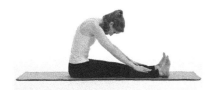

SPINE STRETCH FORWARD
page 98

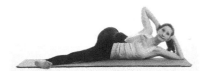

SIDE KICK SERIES: SIDE KICKS
page 100

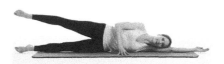

SIDE KICK SERIES: UP & DOWN
page 102

THE HUNDRED

In Level 1, the Hundred is performed with straight legs instead of bent legs (as you did in the modified version on page 50). Straightening the legs makes them heavier, creating more work for the abdominal muscles—which means they'll get stronger! Be sure to perform the Hundred while keeping the belly button pulled to the spine to improve the endurance of the abs. If you feel your abs popping, bend your knees again! Over time, the Hundred will give you flatter abs and a stronger core.

FOCUS: Keep the belly button pulled to the spine, and keep tension out of the neck while inhaling and exhaling fully throughout the exercise.

REPETITIONS: 10 sets of 5 short breaths to inhale and 5 short breaths to exhale, up to the count of 100

VISUALIZATION: Imagine your arms bouncing on a small ball placed under the tops of the arms. Imagine your abs getting flatter and flatter as you progress.

PRECAUTIONS: Avoid this exercise if you have any chronic neck or lower-back pain, or stay with the modified version in the Introductory Program (beginning on page 50).

1. Lie on the mat with your knees bent and feet flat on the floor, legs squeezing together, and arms by your sides. **A** Move to the imprint position. Inhale and lift one leg up into tabletop position, then exhale and lift the other leg up into tabletop. Your femurs should form right angles with your body and your shins. **B**

2. Inhale and tuck the chin slightly, lengthening the back of the neck.

3. Exhale, and use your abdominal muscles to lift your head and shoulders off the mat, maintaining the strong connection between the ribs and hips. **C** Straighten your legs and extend them into a high diagonal. **D**

4. Inhale for 5 short breaths, "sipping" the air in through your nose and pumping your arms up and down slightly.

5. Continue the pumping motion of the arms as you exhale through your mouth for 5 short puffs.

6. Continue for 9 more sets of breaths. Then, as you inhale, curl your head and shoulders off the mat even more.

7. Lower your head and shoulders down to the mat as you exhale. Return one leg and then the other to the mat

A

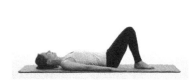

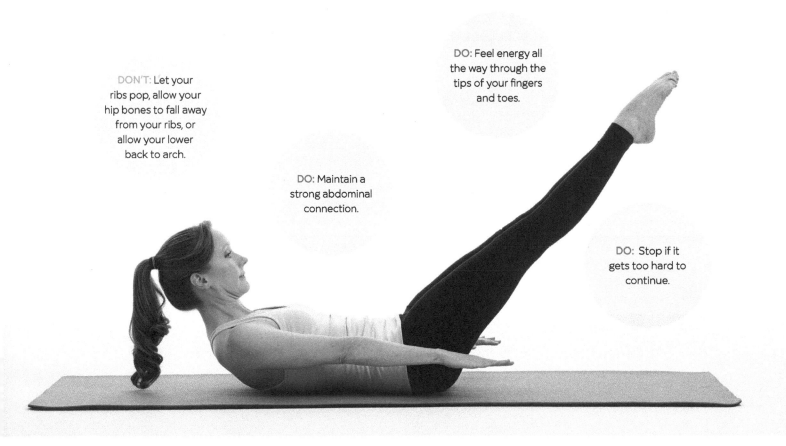

DON'T: Let your ribs pop, allow your hip bones to fall away from your ribs, or allow your lower back to arch.

DO: Maintain a strong abdominal connection.

DO: Feel energy all the way through the tips of your fingers and toes.

DO: Stop if it gets too hard to continue.

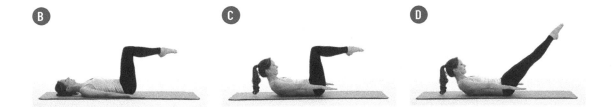

B

C

D

THE ROLL-UP

The Roll-Up is a challenging exercise, especially if you have short legs or a tight lower back. It tends to favor those with naturally flexible spines or long legs. However, anyone can reap the benefits of this exercise; it's excellent for strengthening the abdominals and maintaining the flexibility of the spine.

FOCUS: Execute a smooth roll-up and roll-down without using momentum.

REPETITIONS: 4 to 6

VISUALIZATION: Imagine your spine is a string of pearls that lifts off a dresser one pearl at a time and is placed back down one pearl at a time.

PRECAUTIONS: If you have neck problems, or tightness or discomfort in the lower back, avoid this exercise.

1. Lie on your back with your pelvis and spine neutral, legs together. Reach your arms overhead without popping the ribs. **A**

2. Inhale as you reach your arms to the ceiling and tuck the chin slightly, then lift your head and shoulders off the mat. **B**

3. Exhale as you continue to curl the spine off the mat, one vertebra at a time, **C** lifting the torso until the weight of your body is on your sit bones and the pelvis is neutral, with your spine rounded over your legs. **D**

4. Inhale as you begin to roll the weight backward off the sit bones. **E**

5. Exhale to roll down slowly, vertebra by vertebra, to the start position. **F**

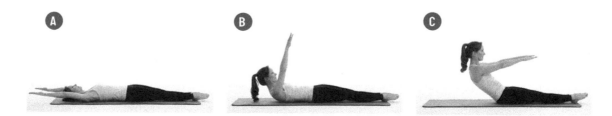

DON'T: Allow momentum to dictate the movement.

DO: Keep your belly button pulled to the spine.

DO: Focus on a smooth, even curve of the spine and maintain fluidity throughout the movement.

DON'T: Let the abdominal muscles pop.

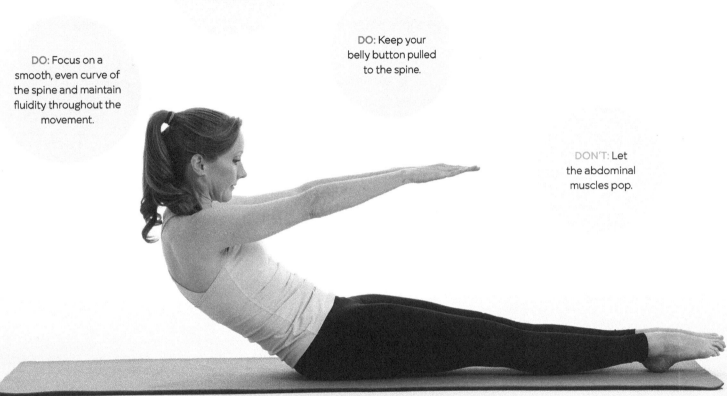

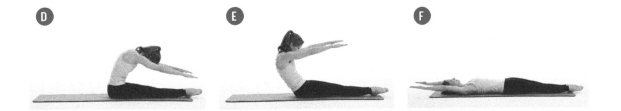

SINGLE-LEG CIRCLES

Single-Leg Circles is another exercise that challenges the stability of the torso against the movement of the legs. You'll do the exercise with both legs straight, if possible. While you may progress to larger circles, the priority in this exercise is the stability of the torso.

FOCUS: Keep the pelvis and spine neutral and stable against the larger circular movement of the legs in the air.

REPETITIONS: 4 to 6 on each side

VISUALIZATION: Imagine a pencil extending out from your big toe, drawing circles on the ceiling.

PRECAUTIONS: If you have lower-back instability, bend the bottom leg for additional support. If you have tight hip flexors, slightly bending the extended leg will alleviate discomfort.

1. Lie on the mat with your legs straight and squeezing together and your arms by your sides. Your pelvis and spine should be neutral, the abdominal muscles pulled in tight. **A**

2. Exhale and lift your right leg into tabletop position. **B** Then extend your knee and point your foot so your leg is reaching to the ceiling at a right angle to the body. **C**

3. While inhaling smoothly, bring your right leg slightly toward your body, across the midline of the body, and then down slightly as if drawing a semicircle on the ceiling. **D**

4. While exhaling smoothly, complete the other half of the circle by moving your leg away from the midline **E** and back up to the top of the circle. **F**

5. Continue in this direction, inhaling for the first half of the circle and exhaling for the second half of the circle, for 4 to 6 repetitions. Reverse the direction, inhaling when your leg moves away from the midline and down, and exhaling when it moves toward the midline and up, for 4 to 6 more repetitions.

6. Repeat with the opposite leg.

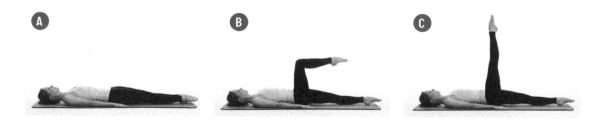

A   **B**   **C**

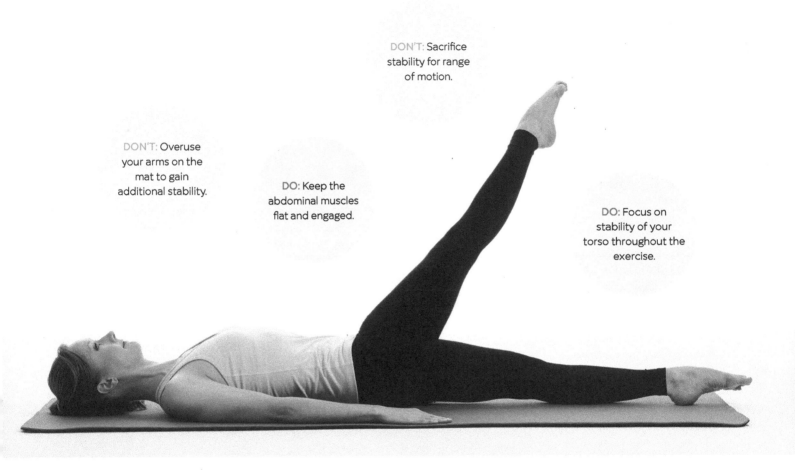

DON'T: Sacrifice stability for range of motion.

DON'T: Overuse your arms on the mat to gain additional stability.

DO: Keep the abdominal muscles flat and engaged.

DO: Focus on stability of your torso throughout the exercise.

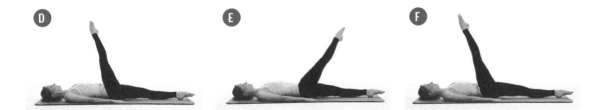

D   E   F

ROLLING LIKE A BALL

This exercise increases spinal flexibility, abdominal strength, and core control. The abdominal muscles are both the accelerator and the brakes in this exercise. Subtle control from the abs is essential to performing the exercise correctly with little momentum.

FOCUS: Maintain a uniform rounding of the spine throughout the exercise so you can roll smoothly without flat spots. Maintain control by using the abdominal muscles so your weight doesn't go to your neck or head and your feet don't touch the mat.

REPETITIONS: 8 to 10

VISUALIZATION: Imagine sitting in the shape of the letter C and rolling in this C throughout the exercise. Imagine contracting the lower fibers of the abdominal muscles more to lift the pelvis when rolling back, and contracting the upper fibers of the abdominal muscles more to lift the head and shoulders when returning.

PRECAUTIONS: If you've been advised to avoid rotation due to lower-back or disc injuries, skip this exercise until you are cleared by a medical professional. Always work in a pain-free range of motion.

1. Sit tall with your weight even on both sit bones, pelvis neutral, knees bent, legs squeezing together, and feet flat on the mat. **A** Contract your abdominal muscles to curl the spine and roll your weight back off the sit bones, gazing at your knees. **B** Then lift your legs one at time to balance on the back of the sit bones, and point your toes. Place your arms gently around your legs, holding your shins. This is the start position. **C**

2. Inhale smoothly and contract the abdominals to roll back, bringing your body weight to the top your shoulder blades (but not onto your neck or head). Continue to gaze at your knees. **D**

3. Exhale smoothly and contract the abdominal muscles more to slide your ribs toward your pelvis to return to the start position and balance on the back of the sit bones without putting your feet down. **E** Repeat.

4. After you finish your reps, place your feet down one at a time.

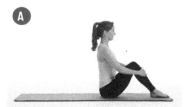

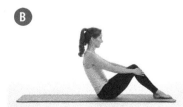

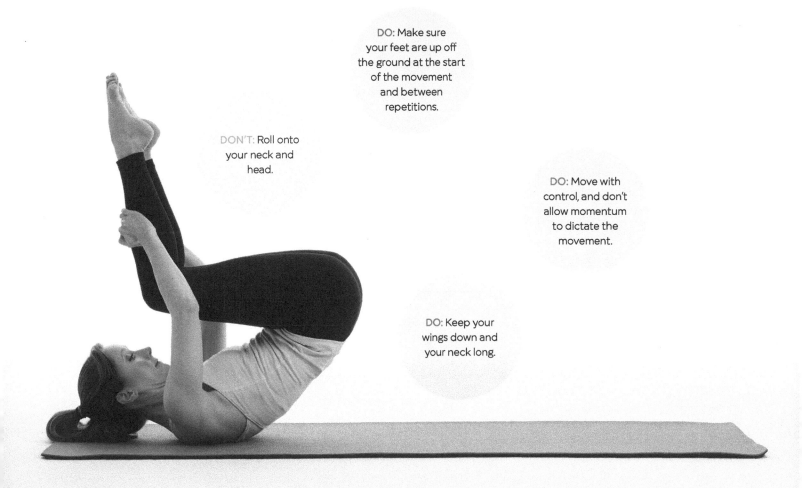

DO: Make sure your feet are up off the ground at the start of the movement and between repetitions.

DON'T: Roll onto your neck and head.

DO: Move with control, and don't allow momentum to dictate the movement.

DO: Keep your wings down and your neck long.

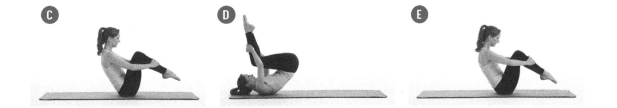

C

D

E

SINGLE-LEG STRETCH

In the Single-Leg Stretch, the hands are no longer supporting the head as they did in the modified version (page 62). Instead, the arms reach toward the feet, which creates more work for the abdominal muscles. In addition, the pace of this version is faster, which challenges your coordination and control.

FOCUS: Keep your abdominal muscles drawn in and flat as your leg reaches as low as possible and your lower back presses into the mat.

REPETITIONS: 8 to 10

VISUALIZATION: Imagine the foot of the extended leg reaching far away from the center. Imagine curling up higher with each repetition.

PRECAUTIONS: If you've been advised to avoid rotation due to lower-back or disc injuries, or if you have a neck injury or neck discomfort, skip this exercise until you are cleared by a medical professional. Always work in a pain-free range of motion.

1. Lie on the mat with both knees bent and feet flat on the floor, legs squeezing together, and arms by your sides. **A** Move to the imprint position. Inhale and lift one leg up into tabletop position, then exhale and lift the other leg up into tabletop. **B** The femurs should form right angles with your body and your shins. Reach your arms toward your ankles with both hands against the outsides of your calves. Lift your head and shoulders off the mat to assume the start position. **C**

2. While inhaling, extend the right leg into a low diagonal (only as low as you can while still maintaining imprint) and reach your arms toward your feet, simultaneously curling up higher off the mat. **D** On the same inhale (similar to the sips in the Hundred, page 80), switch and extend the left leg into a low diagonal (as low as you can while still maintaining imprint), and reach your legs toward your feet while curling up higher. **E**

3. On an exhale, repeat the movement, drawing the left knee to the chest while reaching the right leg as low as you can while still maintaining imprint, and then on the same exhale switch, pulling in the right knee and reaching the left leg out.

4. When you finish your repetitions, bring both legs back to tabletop, lower your head and shoulders to the mat, and then lower the legs one at a time.

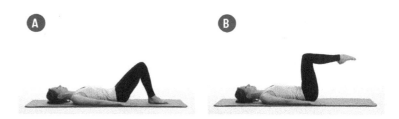

A   **B**

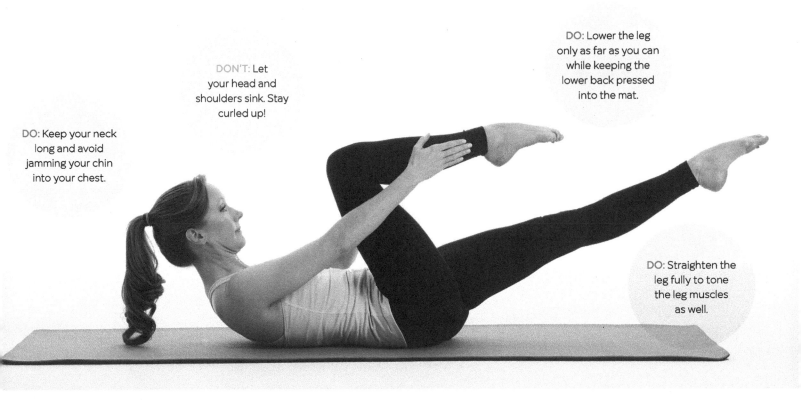

DON'T: Let your head and shoulders sink. Stay curled up!

DO: Keep your neck long and avoid jamming your chin into your chest.

DO: Lower the leg only as far as you can while keeping the lower back pressed into the mat.

DO: Straighten the leg fully to tone the leg muscles as well.

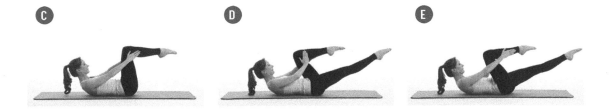

C   D   E

CRISS-CROSS

The Criss-Cross builds on its modified version (page 64) by not only increasing the challenge to the abdominal muscles by lowering the leg but also by increasing the pace of the exercise.

FOCUS: Keep the abdominal muscles drawn in and flat as your leg reaches as low as possible (while still maintaining imprint), and rotate the head, neck, and shoulders as much as possible.

REPETITIONS: 8 to 10

VISUALIZATION: Imagine the foot of the extended leg reaching far away from the center of the body. Imagine curling up higher and increasing rotation with each repetition.

PRECAUTIONS: If you've been advised to avoid rotation due to lower-back or disc injuries, skip this exercise until you are cleared by a medical professional. Always work in a pain-free range of motion.

1. Lie on the mat with both knees bent and feet flat on the floor, legs squeezing together, and arms by your sides. **A** Move to the imprint position. Inhale and lift one leg up into tabletop position, then exhale and lift the other leg up into tabletop. Your femurs should form right angles with your body and your shins. **B** Place both hands behind your head with your thumbs at your hairline and elbows reaching wide. Lift your head and shoulders off the mat to assume the start position. **C**

2. While inhaling, extend your right leg into a low diagonal (as low as you can while still maintaining imprint) and draw your left knee in toward your forehead, simultaneously rotating to the left, reaching your right shoulder to your left knee. **D** On the same inhale (similar to the sips in the Hundred, page 80), switch and rotate right while extending the left leg into a low diagonal (as low as you can while still maintaining imprint) and drawing your right knee closer to your forehead. **E**

3. On an exhale, repeat the movement, drawing the left knee to the chest while reaching the right shoulder to the left knee and extending the right leg toward the floor, **F** then on the same exhale switch, pulling the right knee in with the left leg reaching toward the floor. **G**

4. After you finish your repetitions, bring both legs to tabletop, lower your head and shoulders to the mat, and then lower your legs one at a time.

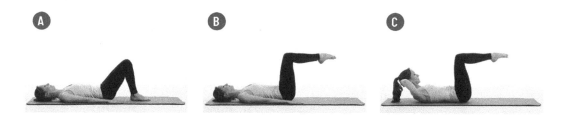

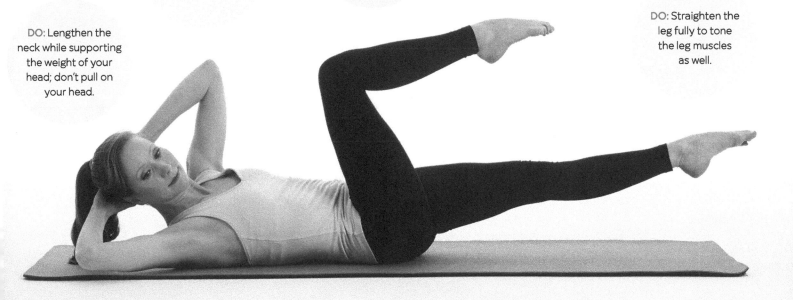

DON'T: Let your head and shoulders sink. Stay curled up!

DO: Keep your elbows wide and rotate your rib cage and shoulders.

DO: Lower the leg only as far as you can while keeping your lower back pressed into the mat.

DO: Lengthen the neck while supporting the weight of your head; don't pull on your head.

DO: Straighten the leg fully to tone the leg muscles as well.

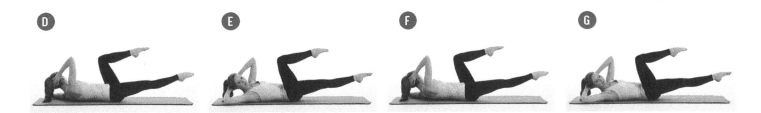

D   E   F   G

DOUBLE-LEG STRETCH, MODIFIED

This move builds on the strength gained in the Single-Leg Stretch (page 88) by extending both legs away from the torso at the same time. This challenges the abdominal muscles and core stabilizers to support the lower back against the weight of both legs.

FOCUS: Maintain a strong imprint as both legs reach out on a diagonal.

REPETITIONS: 6 to 8

VISUALIZATION: Imagine your belly button drawing down as far as possible every time the legs reach away. Imagine being pulled from either direction to keep lengthening.

PRECAUTIONS: If you've been advised to avoid rotation due to lower-back or disc injuries, skip this exercise until you are cleared by a medical professional. Always work in a pain-free range of motion.

1. Lie on the mat with both knees bent and feet flat on the floor, legs squeezing together, and arms by your sides. **A** Move to the imprint position. Inhale and lift one leg up into tabletop position, then exhale and lift the other leg up into tabletop. The femurs should form right angles with your body and your shins. **B** Reach your arms toward your ankles with both hands against the outside of your calves. Lift your head and shoulders off the mat to assume the start position. **C**

2. Exhale and reach your arms overhead by the ears, and extend your legs into a high diagonal. The lower back should not leave the mat. **D**

3. Inhale and bend your knees to return to the start position. **E** Repeat.

4. When you finish your repetitions, lower your head and shoulders to the mat and return one leg and then the other to the mat.

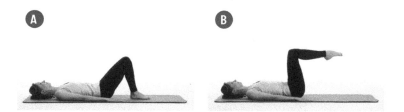

A   **B**

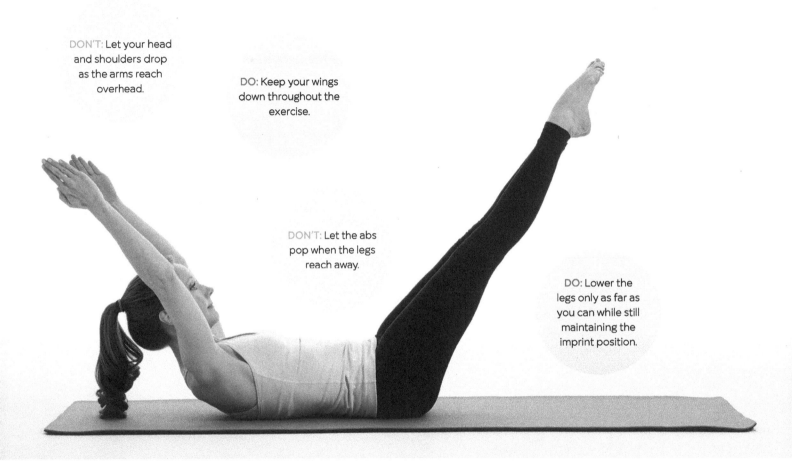

DON'T: Let your head and shoulders drop as the arms reach overhead.

DO: Keep your wings down throughout the exercise.

DON'T: Let the abs pop when the legs reach away.

DO: Lower the legs only as far as you can while still maintaining the imprint position.

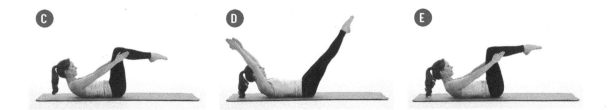

C

D

E

BREAST STROKE

The Breast Stroke improves posture by strengthening the muscles of the upper back, increasing flexibility of the upper spine, and stabilizing the core. It also helps tone the muscles of the back of the arms to create strong, lean, shapely muscles.

FOCUS: Isolate the muscles of the upper back without involving the muscles of the lower back, all while keeping the abs flat and engaged.

REPETITIONS: 4 to 6

VISUALIZATION: As you reach your arms overhead, imagine that you are a torpedo. Then, as your arms sweep around and your spine extends, imagine that your heart is reaching forward toward the wall in front of you.

PRECAUTIONS: If you have any diagnosed spinal conditions, especially in the cervical spine, consult your doctors before attempting this exercise. If you experience lower-back pain, you may want to place a cushion under your hip bones.

1. Lie on your stomach with your legs shoulder-width apart. Your pelvis and spine should be neutral, your legs together and parallel. Place your hands on the floor, comfortably just outside of your shoulders with your elbows bent. **A**

2. Inhale to pull your belly button to your spine and lengthen through the top of your head.

3. As you exhale, reach your arms straight overhead and slightly lift your torso so that you're hovering just over the mat. **B**

4. On a long, continuous inhale, sweep your arms around wide and to the sides **C** until they are by your thighs, simultaneously extending your spine to lift your head and shoulders off the mat. **D** Repeat.

5. When you finish your repetitions, slowly lower everything down to the start position.

A

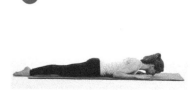

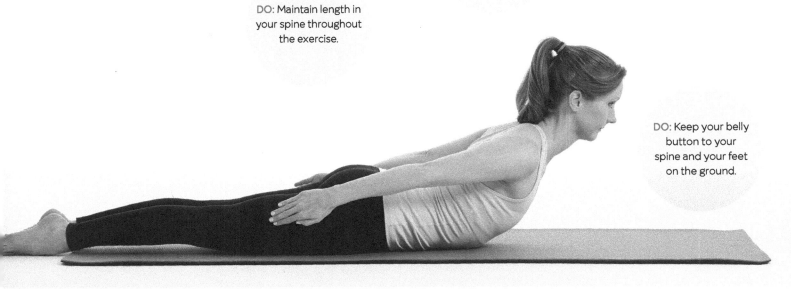

DON'T: Over-extend your neck! (There should be no wrinkles on your neck as you perform the exercise.)

DO: Maintain length in your spine throughout the exercise.

DO: Keep your belly button to your spine and your feet on the ground.

B

C

D

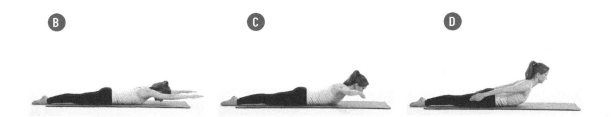

SPINE TWIST

Building on the Introductory Program Spine Twist (page 56), the Level 1 Spine Twist is performed on the mat with your legs straight. This version further increases spinal mobility in rotation while improving core stability, which is important for everyday activities as well as sports.

FOCUS: Maintain upright posture with your legs straight while you rotate to your full range of motion.

REPETITIONS: 4 to 6

VISUALIZATION: Imagine your spine is a barber shop pole, continuously spiraling upward and getting taller.

PRECAUTIONS: If you've been advised to avoid rotation due to lower-back or disc injuries, skip this exercise until you are cleared by a medical professional. Always work in a pain-free range of motion.

1. Sit on top of your sit bones with your legs as straight as possible and your pelvis and spine neutral. Ideally, your legs are squeezing together, but if you experience discomfort, separate the legs slightly. Reach your arms out to the sides to where you can still see your fingers in your peripheral vision. Pull in your abdominal muscles, slide your wings down, and sit as tall as possible, lengthening through the top of your head. **A**

2. As with the modified Spine Twist (page 56), take 3 inhales in succession as if you are taking 3 sniffs of air through the nose to fill your lungs. While inhaling, twist your spine to the left. At the end range of your rotation, continue inhaling with 2 more sniffs to gently increase your range of rotation. Turn your head to the left as well, looking toward your left fingers. **B**

3. While exhaling smoothly, untwist the spine to return to the start position. Make sure that your shoulders are down and your abdominal muscles are flat. **C**

4. Repeat the movement to the right. **D**

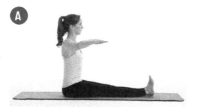

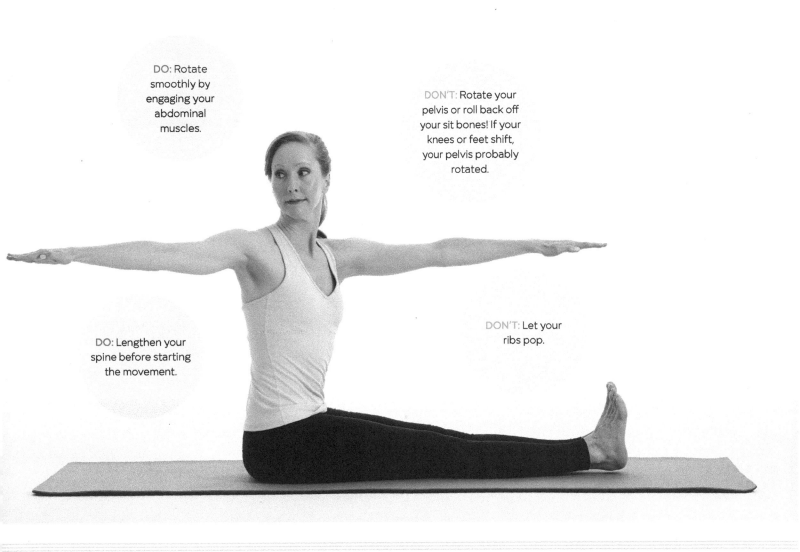

DO: Rotate smoothly by engaging your abdominal muscles.

DON'T: Rotate your pelvis or roll back off your sit bones! If your knees or feet shift, your pelvis probably rotated.

DO: Lengthen your spine before starting the movement.

DON'T: Let your ribs pop.

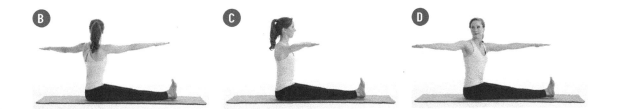

B

C

D

SPINE STRETCH FORWARD

This exercise helps build awareness of the muscles on the front and back of the spine that control both movement and stability. Over time, the Spine Stretch Forward will help you cultivate both a flexible spine and improved posture.

FOCUS: Move your spine one vertebra at a time in order to control the movement in both directions.

REPETITIONS: 4 to 6

VISUALIZATION: Imagine that your spine is a piece of tape on a wall—you peel it off the wall slowly and then press it back to the wall from the bottom up.

PRECAUTIONS: Individuals with osteoporosis or an exaggerated kyphosis of the thoracic spine should avoid this exercise. If you've had any herniated discs, proceed with caution. If you've been advised to avoid forward bending of the spine, avoid this exercise.

1. Sit on your mat with your legs outstretched and feet shoulder-width apart. Your pelvis and spine should be neutral. Rest your hands on the tops of your thighs. **A**

2. Inhale and pull your belly button to your spine, lengthening through the top of your head.

3. Exhale to roll down one vertebra at a time, starting by tucking the chin and then rounding through the upper back, **B** mid back, **C** and lower back. Keep your pelvis neutral. **D**

4. Inhale in this position, maintaining the abdominal connection and the shape of the spine.

5. Exhale to bring the torso back to vertical, rolling the spine up one vertebra at a time. **E**

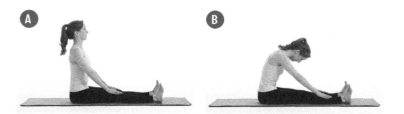

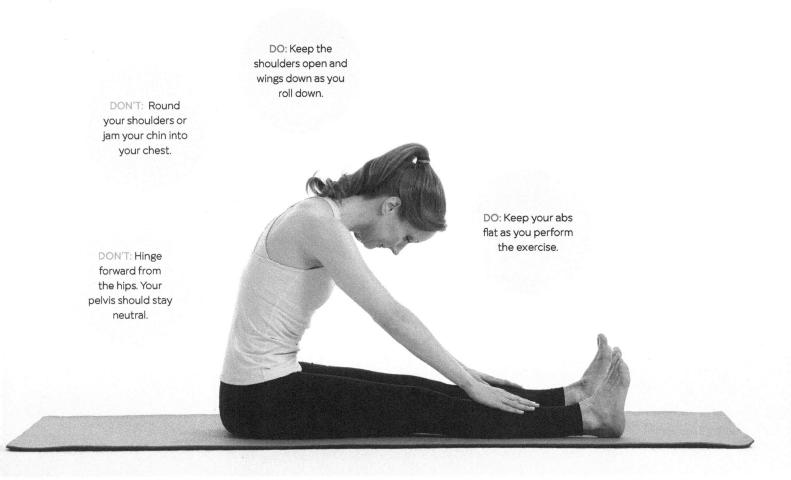

DON'T: Round your shoulders or jam your chin into your chest.

DON'T: Hinge forward from the hips. Your pelvis should stay neutral.

DO: Keep the shoulders open and wings down as you roll down.

DO: Keep your abs flat as you perform the exercise.

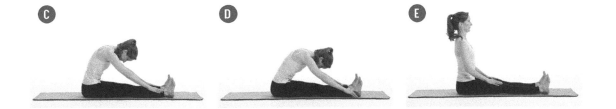

C

D

E

SIDE KICK SERIES

You begin all Side Kick exercises by lying on your side. We introduce two versions here in Level 1, and you'll find three more in Level 2 (beginning on page 107). The kicks are more stabilization exercises than flexibility exercises.

SIDE KICKS

For this exercise, the forward-and-back swinging motion of the leg is secondary to the stability of the spine.

FOCUS: Keep your spine and pelvis neutral and stable while the top leg is swinging either forward or back.

REPETITIONS: 6 to 10 on each side

VISUALIZATION: Imagine that your spine is a steel rod from which your leg swings freely like a pendulum.

PRECAUTIONS: If you have tight hamstrings or hip flexors, modify your range of motion as necessary.

1. Lie on one side with your hips stacked and your legs straight and at a 30- to 40-degree angle in front of you. Prop your head up on your bottom hand with the elbow bent, and place your other hand behind your head. Your pelvis and spine should be neutral. **A**

2. Inhale to lengthen through the spine, and pull your belly button to your spine.

3. As you exhale, lift the top leg up to hip height. **B**

4. Inhale for 2 breaths, kicking the top leg forward toward your chest and pulsing the leg twice. **C**

5. On 1 smooth and long exhale, press that same leg back as far as you can while still maintaining a neutral pelvis and spine. **D**

A

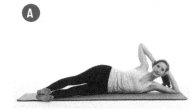

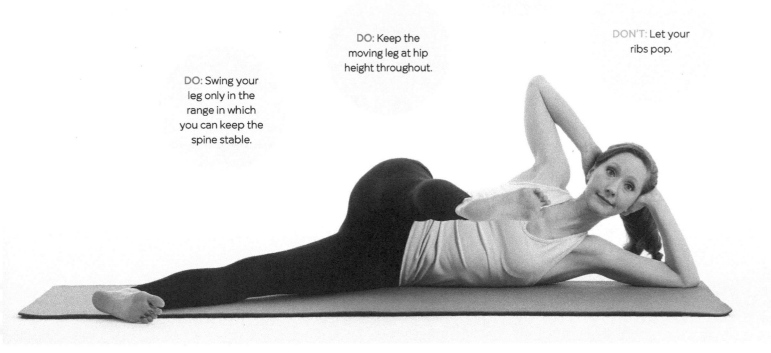

DON'T: Collapse the spine or allow your pelvis to tip back when the leg moves forward.

DO: Keep the moving leg at hip height throughout.

DON'T: Let your ribs pop.

DO: Swing your leg only in the range in which you can keep the spine stable.

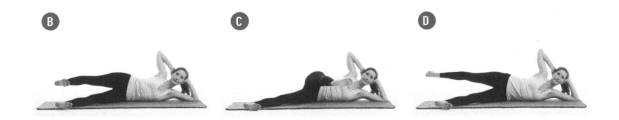

B

C

D

SIDE KICK SERIES

UP & DOWN

The Up & Down exercise works on strengthening the muscles of your outer hip and leg, all the while stabilizing the spine and toning the abs.

FOCUS: Keep your spine, pelvis, and hips neutral as the top leg works.

REPETITIONS: 6 to 10 on each side

VISUALIZATION: Imagine that your spine is a steel rod, impervious to movement regardless of what the legs are doing.

PRECAUTIONS: If you have a tight lower back, you may need to flex the hips slightly during this exercise. If you have neck pain, you might want to place a pillow under your head.

1. Lie on one side with your hips stacked and your feet in line with your hips. Your body will be in a straight line. Extend your bottom arm straight overhead, and allow your head to rest on it, or if it is more comfortable, bend your bottom arm and rest your head in your hand.. The top arm is bent, with your hand resting on the floor. Your pelvis and spine should be neutral, with your abs pulling in firmly. **A**

2. Inhale to lengthen through the spine, and pull your belly button to your spine. Simultaneously, lift the top leg slightly higher than hip height but not so high that your top hip hikes up to your ribs. Keep the knee facing forward. **B**

3. As you exhale, flex your foot **C** and then lower the leg down to the start position. **D** Repeat 6 to 10 times.

4. Repeat on the other side.

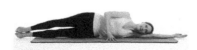

A

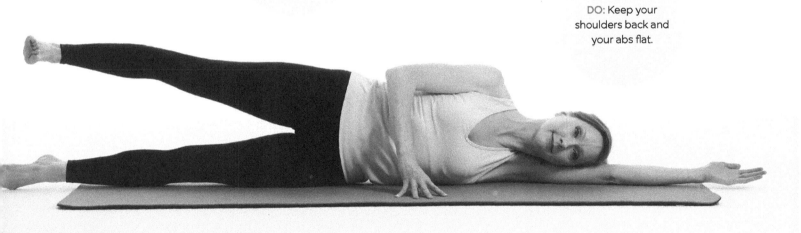

DO: Keep energy in your legs.

DO: Keep both knees pointing straight forward.

DON'T: Allow your top hip to hike up as the top leg lifts.

DO: Keep your shoulders back and your abs flat.

B

C

D

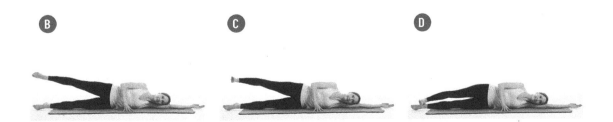

ASSESSING YOUR PROGRESS

By the end of the Level 1 Program, your strength, range of motion, body awareness, and confidence have all increased! Be proud of your progress, and remember that successful completion of Level 1 doesn't mean that you can perform each and every exercise perfectly. Every *body* is different, so be kind to yourself when you take note of what still needs work. The point is that you understand, acknowledge, and embrace the uniqueness of your body and your needs.

To that end, be honest and compassionate with yourself in this self-assessment. If you answer "yes" to all of these questions, move ahead to Level 2. If you answer "no" to a few, take a bit more time in Level 1. Remember, as we've said before, Pilates is a marathon, not a sprint. If you need to take one or two more weeks in Level 1, you will be stronger and better for it in the long run.

1. Can you roll through the spine smoothly? If you have flat spots, do you know how to adjust your practice to keep yourself comfortable?

2. Can you stabilize your pelvis in neutral against the movement of the legs, as in Single-Leg Circles (page 84) or Side Kicks (page 100)? If you cannot keep your torso still with full range of motion, can you do so if you modify the range of motion?

3. Do you understand your own limits? Do you know when your abs are popping or your lower back is lifting when you lower your legs?

4. Do you have the abdominal endurance to execute exercises such as the Hundred (page 80) and Rolling Like a Ball (page 86)?

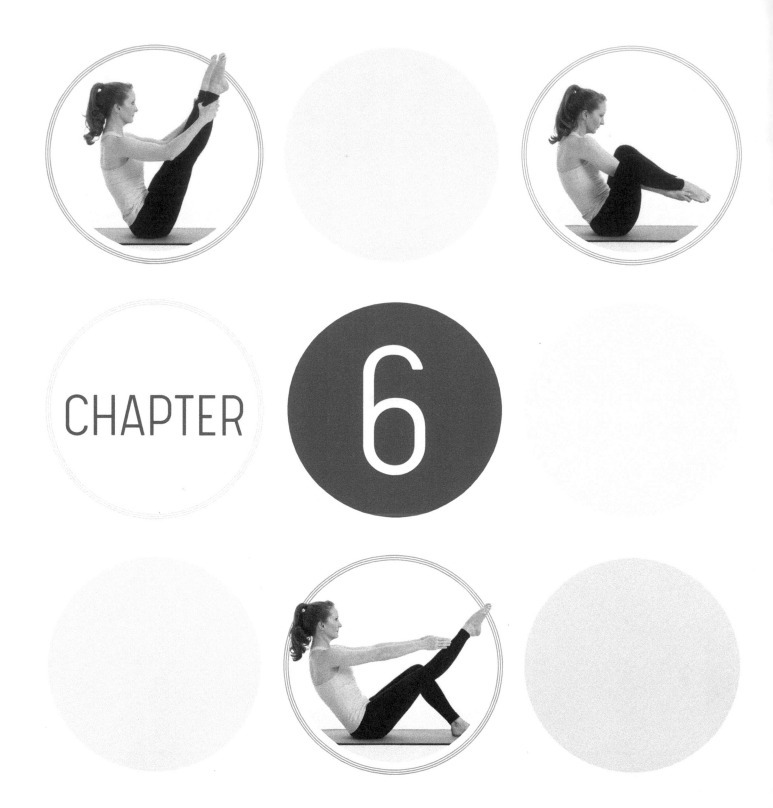

CHAPTER 6

LEVEL 2 PROGRAM

CONGRATULATIONS—YOU'VE REACHED LEVEL 2! By this stage, you have increased your core strength, range of motion, and spinal flexibility. You've also developed an awareness and understanding of your own body and its unique strengths and weaknesses. You are ready to take on more challenging exercises. In this program, expect your abs, core, legs, and arms to become even stronger. Your flexibility and body awareness will continue to improve, too!

LEVEL 2 SEQUENCE

With the Level 2 Sequence, we continue to build upon the technique and strength gains made in the Introductory and Level 1 Sequences. The Level 2 Sequence should not be tacked on to the end of the Level 1 Sequence; rather, the full versions of certain exercises replace their modified counterparts, and new exercises appear as well. Continue to practice and perfect the Shoulder Bridge and Mermaid Stretch, even though they do not have more advanced versions in Level 2.

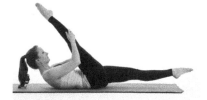

SINGLE STRAIGHT-LEG STRETCH
(SCISSORS)
page 110

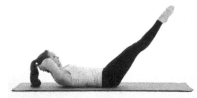

DOUBLE STRAIGHT-LEG STRETCH
(LOWER & LIFT)
page 112

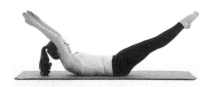

DOUBLE-LEG STRETCH
page 114

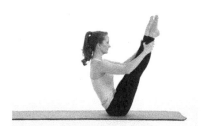

OPEN-LEG ROCKER
page 116

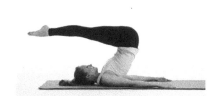

THE ROLLOVER
page 118

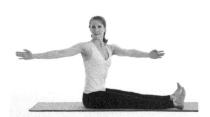

THE SAW
page 120

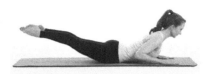

SWAN DIVE 2, MODIFIED
page 122

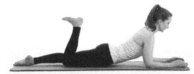

SINGLE-LEG KICK
page 124

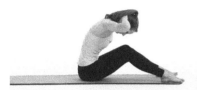

NECK PULL, MODIFIED
page 126

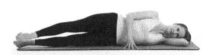

SIDE KICK SERIES: CIRCLES
page 128

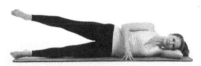

SIDE KICK SERIES: STAGGERED LEGS
page 130

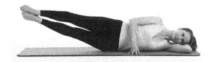

SIDE KICK SERIES: DOUBLE-LEG LIFT
page 132

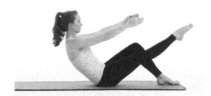

THE TEASER, MODIFIED
page 134

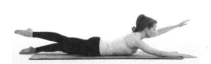

SWIMMING, MODIFIED
page 136

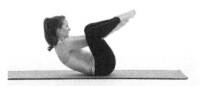

THE SEAL
page 138

SINGLE STRAIGHT-LEG STRETCH (SCISSORS)

The Single Straight-Leg Stretch builds on the Single-Leg Stretch (page 88) by challenging the abdominal muscles with the longer lever of the straight legs. In addition to building abdominal strength and endurance, this exercise increases flexibility of the hamstrings.

FOCUS: Maintain an imprint position of the spine against the large range of motion of the legs.

REPETITIONS: 8 to 10

VISUALIZATION: Imagine your legs are tracing the full arc of a rainbow as they alternate reaching toward and away from the torso. Envision each leg getting longer and longer as the rainbow is traced.

PRECAUTIONS: If you've been advised to avoid rotation due to lower-back or disc injuries, skip this exercise until you are cleared by a medical professional. Always work in a pain-free range of motion.

1. Lie on your back on the mat with both knees bent and feet flat on the floor, legs squeezing together, and your arms by your sides. **A** Move to the imprint position. Inhale and lift one leg up into tabletop position, then exhale and lift the other leg up into tabletop. **B** Extend your knees so both legs are reaching up to the ceiling, forming a right angle to your torso. Point your feet. **C** Lift your head and shoulders off the mat and lift your arms slightly, reaching the arms long out in front of you to assume the start position. **D**

2. Exhale and open your legs like a pair of scissors: Lower the right leg toward your body, guiding the leg with your hands, and extend the left leg away toward the ground. Then exhale again with a slight, gentle pulse at the end range to reach both legs farther, slightly increasing the stretch. **E**

3. Inhale to lift both legs back to pass through the start position. **F**

4. Exhale and switch and scissor the legs the opposite way, lowering the left leg toward the body, guiding the leg with your hands, while reaching the right leg away. Exhale again and pulse once at the end range.

5. After you finish your reps, reach both legs to the ceiling, then bend your knees, lower your head and shoulders to the mat, and lower each leg one at a time.

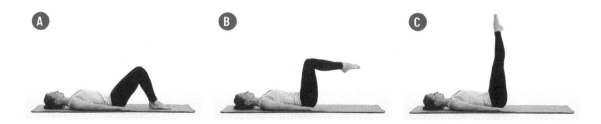

A   **B**   **C**

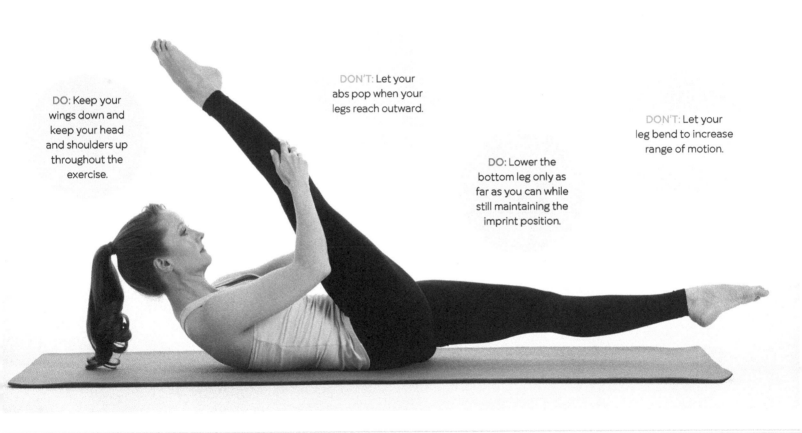

DO: Keep your wings down and keep your head and shoulders up throughout the exercise.

DON'T: Let your abs pop when your legs reach outward.

DON'T: Let your leg bend to increase range of motion.

DO: Lower the bottom leg only as far as you can while still maintaining the imprint position.

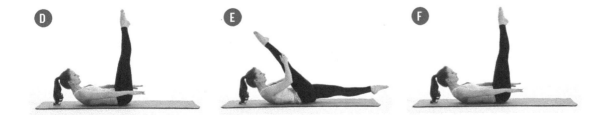

D

E

F

DOUBLE STRAIGHT-LEG STRETCH (LOWER & LIFT)

The Double Straight-Leg Stretch, or "Lower & Lift," challenges the abdominal muscles to hold the pelvis and spine in imprint against the weight of the straight legs lowering toward the mat.

FOCUS: Maintain a strong imprint position with flat abdominal muscles as the legs lower to the mat as far as you can while keeping the movement controlled.

REPETITIONS: 8 to 10

VISUALIZATION: Imagine a heavy weight on the abs that keeps your lower back pressed to the mat and prevents the abs from pushing out from the spine.

PRECAUTIONS: If you have lower-back or disc injuries, or if you have been advised against flexing the spine, skip this exercise until you are cleared by a medical professional. Always work in a pain-free range of motion. If you have neck injuries or neck pain, keep your head resting on the mat during this exercise.

1. Lie on the mat with both knees bent and feet flat on the floor, legs squeezing together, and arms by your sides. Ⓐ Move to the imprint position. Inhale and lift one leg up into tabletop position, then exhale and lift the other leg up into tabletop. Ⓑ Extend your knees so both legs are reaching to the ceiling, forming a right angle to your torso. Rotate your femurs so your knees face out to the sides. Squeeze your legs together and point your feet. Ⓒ Place your hands behind your head with your thumbs at your hairline, and then lift your head and shoulders off the mat to assume the start position. Ⓓ

2. On a smooth, long exhale, lower your legs only as low as you can while still keeping your lower back pressed to the mat and the abdominal muscles flat. Ⓔ

3. Inhale and lift the legs back to the start position. Ⓕ Repeat.

4. After you finish your reps, bend both knees, lower your head and shoulders to the mat, and place your feet down on the mat, one at a time.

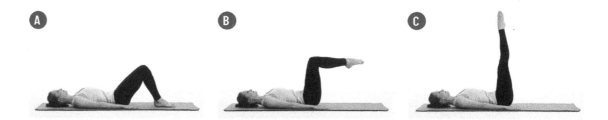

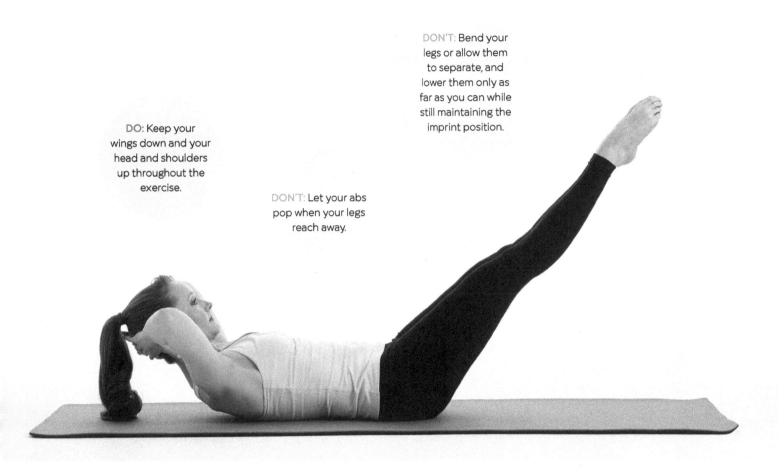

DO: Keep your wings down and your head and shoulders up throughout the exercise.

DON'T: Let your abs pop when your legs reach away.

DON'T: Bend your legs or allow them to separate, and lower them only as far as you can while still maintaining the imprint position.

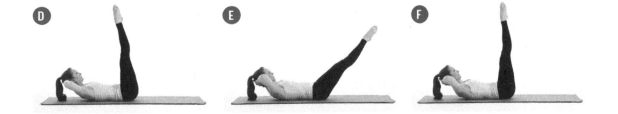

D E F

DOUBLE-LEG STRETCH

In Level 2, the Double-Leg Stretch reaches the legs on a lower diagonal than in the modified version (page 92). The legs are lowered as far you can while still maintaining the imprint position. This is especially challenging with the arms reaching overhead.

FOCUS: Keep the abdominal muscles pulled in and flat and your spine pressed into the mat while your arms and legs reach away from the torso.

REPETITIONS: 6 to 8

VISUALIZATION: Imagine that your body is an accordion being played and that both phases of this movement—reaching the arms and legs away AND pulling the legs and arms back in—require equal amounts of energy. Envision being pulled from each direction when the arms and legs reach away.

PRECAUTIONS: If you've been advised to avoid flexing the spine due to lower-back or disc injuries, skip this exercise until you are cleared by a medical professional. Always work in a pain-free range of motion. If you have neck injuries or neck pain, keep your head resting on the mat.

1. Lie on the mat with both knees bent, legs squeezing together, arms by your sides. **A** Move to the imprint position. Inhale and lift one leg up into tabletop position, then exhale and lift the other leg up into tabletop. Your femurs should form right angles with your body and your shins. **B** Reach the arms toward your ankles with both hands pressing against the outsides of your calves. Lift your head and shoulders off the mat to assume the start position. **C**

2. Exhale and reach your arms straight overhead by your ears and extend your legs into a low diagonal, as low as you can while still maintaining an imprint position. **D**

3. Inhale, bend your knees to pass through tabletop, and circle your arms out wide and to your knees to pull the knees toward your chest. Reach your hands toward your ankles. **E** Repeat.

4. When you've finished your repetitions, lower the head and shoulders down to the mat. Return one leg, then the other, down to the mat.

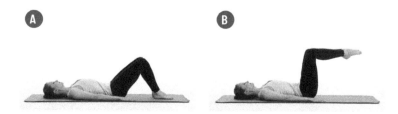

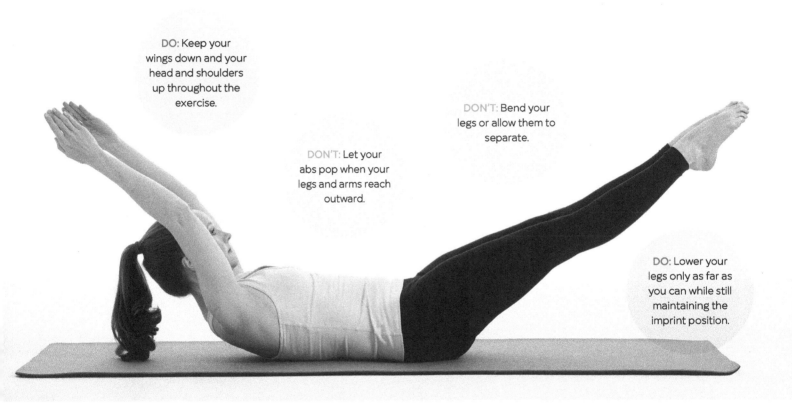

DO: Keep your wings down and your head and shoulders up throughout the exercise.

DON'T: Let your abs pop when your legs and arms reach outward.

DON'T: Bend your legs or allow them to separate.

DO: Lower your legs only as far as you can while still maintaining the imprint position.

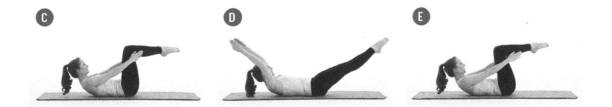

OPEN-LEG ROCKER

In this exercise, the knees are ideally straight, or bent as needed to accommodate hamstring flexibility or core control. The belly is scooped to the spine, but the upper back, shoulders, head, and neck maintain neutral positions, as if you were seated or standing.

FOCUS: Roll smoothly to your mid shoulder blades and then back to the sacrum without changing the shape of your spine or the height of your legs.

REPETITIONS: 8 to 10

VISUALIZATION: Although the shape looks more like a V, imagine your body is forming a U, with your lower back rounded but your upper back neutral and lengthened.

PRECAUTIONS: If you've been advised to avoid rotation due to lower-back or disc injuries, skip this exercise until you are cleared by a medical professional. Always work in a pain-free range of motion.

1. Sit tall with your weight even on both sit bones, your pelvis neutral, knees bent, legs squeezing together, and feet flat on the mat. **A** Contract your abdominal muscles to curl the spine and roll your weight back off the sit bones, gazing at your knees. **B** Then lift your legs one at time and hold your legs outside the calves to balance on the back of the sit bones. Point your toes. **C** Maintaining balance, extend your legs to the ceiling and open them shoulder-width apart while lengthening your upper back. This is the start position. **D**

2. Modification: If the straight-leg position proves too challenging (which is likely if you have long legs!), instead of straightening your legs fully, bend your knees so your shins are parallel to the floor. Hold the outsides of the shins and maintain this position throughout the exercise. Over time, your legs will become straighter and straighter as your hamstring flexibility increases.

3. Inhale smoothly; deepen the contraction of the abdominals to curl your upper back as you contract your lower abdominals more to roll back to the top of your shoulder blades, but not onto your neck or head. If the legs are straight, don't let them bend or touch the floor! If the legs are bent, don't let them straighten. Keep gazing at the knees. **E**

4. Exhale smoothly and contract the abdominal muscles more to slide your ribs toward your pelvis to return to the start position, lengthening your upper spine again. Balance without putting down your feet. **F** After your reps, place your feet down, one at a time.

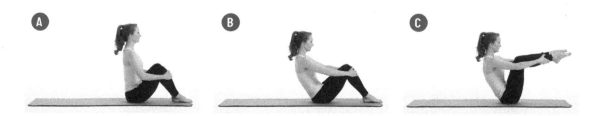

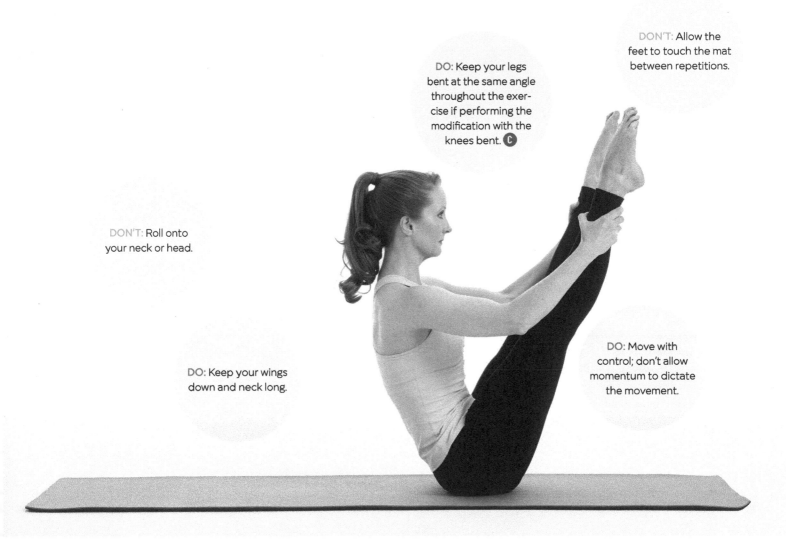

DON'T: Allow the feet to touch the mat between repetitions.

DO: Keep your legs bent at the same angle throughout the exercise if performing the modification with the knees bent. C

DON'T: Roll onto your neck or head.

DO: Keep your wings down and neck long.

DO: Move with control; don't allow momentum to dictate the movement.

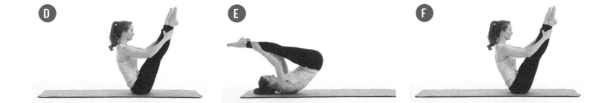

D

E

F

THE ROLLOVER

The Rollover strengthens the muscles of the lower abdomen to lift the hips fully off the mat and take the legs over the head, increasing spinal and hamstring flexibility as well.

FOCUS: Maintain flat abs and control throughout the full exercise. The exercise should be performed with absolutely no momentum and no excessive weight in the arms.

REPETITIONS: 2 to 3 in each direction

VISUALIZATION: Imagine the body creating the shape of a hairpin as it rolls over and then unrolls.

PRECAUTIONS: Individuals with lower-back problems should start with the hips elevated slightly or eliminate the exercise altogether. Individuals with neck problems should continue to do the modified rollover.

1. Lie on the mat with both knees bent and feet flat on the floor, legs squeezing together, and your arms by your sides. **A** Move to the imprint position. Inhale and lift one leg up into tabletop position, then exhale and lift the other leg up into tabletop. Your femurs should form right angles with your body and your shins. **B**

2. Exhale and straighten the knees as you stretch your legs into a high diagonal while maintaining the imprint position. **C** Inhale to engage the abs, and reach both legs to the ceiling (90 degrees). **D**

3. Exhale and contract the abdominal muscles to lift the hips off the mat, sending your toes to the ceiling and then overhead toward the wall behind you. The weight of your body will be between the shoulder blades. Legs are parallel to the floor. **E**

4. Inhale and open the legs shoulder-width apart, then flex your feet.

5. Exhale and roll down, one vertebra at a time, until the pelvis is on the mat and your legs have returned to a high diagonal. **F**

6. Inhale to close the legs, and repeat the exercise 2 more times. On the last repetition, leave the legs separated shoulder-width apart.

7. Then reverse the movement of the legs: Everything stays the same, except now the legs will be separated shoulder-width apart when you roll over and will close when you roll down.

8. After you finish your reps, roll the hips down to the mat.

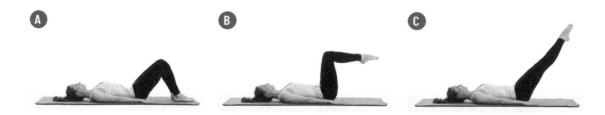

A   **B**   **C**

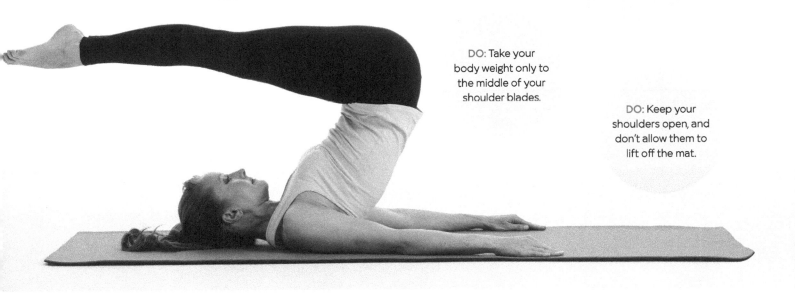

DO: Keep your abs flat.

DON'T: Allow momentum to dictate the movement.

DO: Take your body weight only to the middle of your shoulder blades.

DO: Keep your shoulders open, and don't allow them to lift off the mat.

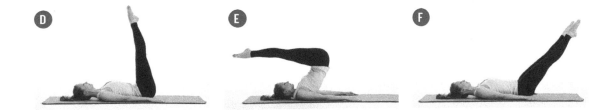

D

E

F

THE SAW

Spine Twist (page 96) + Spine Stretch Forward (page 98) = Saw! The Saw increases flexibility of the spine in forward bending (flexion) and rotation, which is very important for everyday tasks. It also helps develop awareness of the muscles around the spine, as well as the abdominal muscles. The Saw will keep you mindful of excellent posture, help strengthen your core for functional tasks, and provide a great stretch for the lower back.

FOCUS: Maintain the rotation of the spine even when the spine flexes forward, and keep the pelvis in a neutral position.

REPETITIONS: 4 to 6 on each side

VISUALIZATION: First, imagine that you are a barber shop pole, and as you rotate, your spine gets longer. Then, you become the water coming out of a water fountain, traveling up before moving over and down.

PRECAUTIONS: Individuals with osteoporosis or an exaggerated kyphosis of the thoracic spine should avoid this exercise, as should individuals with any history of herniated discs.

1. Sit on the mat with your legs outstretched in front of you, shoulder-width apart, feet flexed. Your pelvis and spine should be neutral, your arms outstretched to the sides at shoulder height, and your palms facing forward, still visible in your peripheral vision. If your hamstrings or hip flexors are tight, sit on a small cushion in order to get the pelvis in a neutral and vertical position. **A**

2. Inhale as you rotate the rib cage and shoulders to the right. **B**

3. Exhale to tuck the chin slightly, and continue to exhale to roll down, one vertebra at a time, scooping the abs. Reach your left arm to the outside of your right foot, and rotate your right arm so that the thumb points toward the floor. The pelvis stays vertical. **C**

4. Then, maintaining the spinal rotation, inhale as you roll up, one vertebra at a time, until your torso is vertical. Both palms face forward. **D**

5. Exhale as you rotate the rib cage and shoulders back to the start position. **E** Repeat on the other side. **F G H**

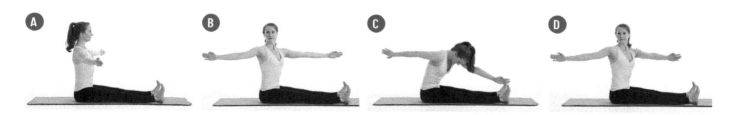

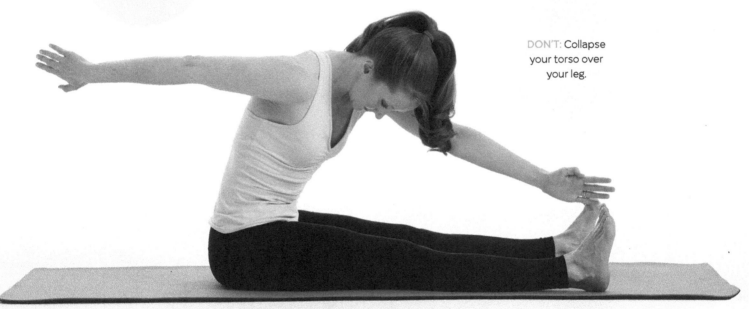

DO: Keep your wings down, and keep length in the spine even while rotating and flexing.

DO: Maintain flat abs throughout the exercise.

DON'T: Collapse your torso over your leg.

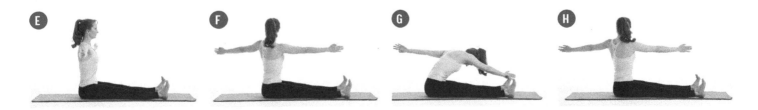

E F G H

SWAN DIVE 2, MODIFIED

The Swan Dive is an advanced exercise that challenges spinal flexibility, core strength, and body awareness. Both this exercise and the Swan Dive, Modified (page 70) are building blocks for Joseph Pilates's advanced classical Swan Dive. This version builds on the foundation developed in the modified version by further challenging the hip extensors (the glutes and hamstrings), as well as the muscles of the abs and back, to maintain the fully extended position of the whole body.

FOCUS: Move the spine into its own full, uniform extension with no pain or discomfort. Maintain core control as the whole body rocks slowly forward and back.

REPETITIONS: 4 to 6

VISUALIZATION: Imagine that you are the bottom of a rocking horse, and that your shape does not change as you rock slowly forward and back.

PRECAUTIONS: Individuals with exaggerated kyphosis of the thoracic spine may need to modify. Individuals with exaggerated lordosis of the lumbar spine or lower-back pain may need to reduce the range of motion or avoid the exercise altogether. If you've been advised against back bending (extension of the spine), avoid this exercise.

1. Lie on your stomach and separate your legs shoulder-width apart. The pelvis and spine should be neutral, and your legs rotated so your knees are pointing to the sides. Place your hands on the floor, comfortably just outside the shoulders with your elbows bent. Pull your belly button to the spine. **A**

2. Inhale and press into the hands to lift your head, shoulders, and as much of the rib cage as your flexibility allows off the mat. Your elbows may or may not straighten fully. **B**

3. As you exhale, contract the glutes to support the weight of your legs as they lift off the mat, simultaneously bending the elbows to maintain the shape of the entire body, **C** and rock the weight of your body forward to the torso. **D**

4. Inhale as you straighten your elbows and engage the muscles of the upper back to lift the torso and restore the body back to the "swan" position with the legs on the ground. **E** Repeat steps 3 and 4.

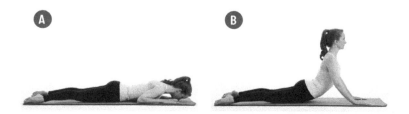

DON'T: Allow the shoulders to lift or hunch.

DON'T: Drop your chin as you bend your elbows to rock your body forward.

DO: Engage the glutes to maintain the position of your legs.

DO: Keep your belly button pulled to the spine throughout the movement.

DO: Keep your wings down, and keep tension out of the neck

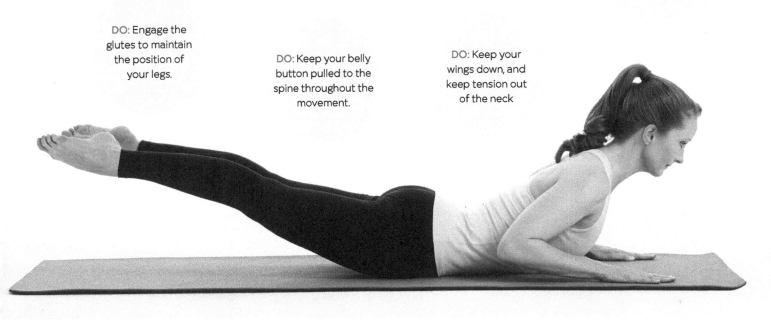

C   D   E

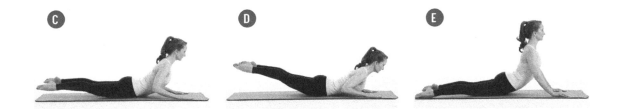

SINGLE-LEG KICK

The Single-Leg Kick helps stabilize the pelvis and spine against the movement of the legs, augmenting core strength and control. It also improves flexibility in the quads and strengthens the shoulder girdle.

FOCUS: Keep the top part of the leg—from the hip bone to the knee—flush on the mat while you bend your knee to bring your heel toward your seat.

REPETITIONS: 6 to 8 on each side

VISUALIZATION: Imagine the abdominal muscles pulling in so much that they—not your elbows—support the weight of your torso. Envision your leg getting longer with each repetition.

PRECAUTIONS: If you've been advised against back bending, limit spinal extension and support the position with the abdominal muscles. If you have knee injuries, be careful to move only in a pain-free range of motion, and skip this exercise if you still experience pain. If you have especially tight quads, you may find this exercise challenging; work in a pain-free range of motion and gradually you will feel improvements.

1. Lie on your stomach with your legs straight and squeezing together and your toes pointed. Place your elbows on the mat directly under your shoulders so that the upper body is propped up but the pubic bone is still touching the mat. Your hip bones will be slightly off the mat. Engage your glutes to help prevent the lower back from arching. Engage your abdominal muscles, lengthen your neck and spine, and slide your shoulders down your back. **A**

2. Modification: If this position is uncomfortable, lie on your stomach with your hands under your forehead, keeping the pelvis and spine neutral.

3. On an exhale, bend the knee of your right leg to kick the heel to the right buttock with a pointed foot, **B** then on a second exhale pulse at the end range for a second kick with a flexed foot. **C**

4. Inhale smoothly, then straighten your right leg, point your toe, **D** and lengthen the leg back down to the mat. **E**

5. Repeat with the left leg.

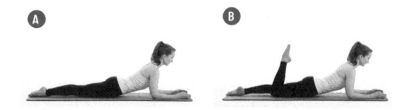

DON'T: Hyperextend your neck.

DO: Keep your wings down.

DO: Keep your pubic bone on the mat and your torso stable as the knee bends and straightens.

DO: Keep the abdominal muscles pulled in and up throughout the exercise.

DON'T: Allow your pelvis and spine to move.

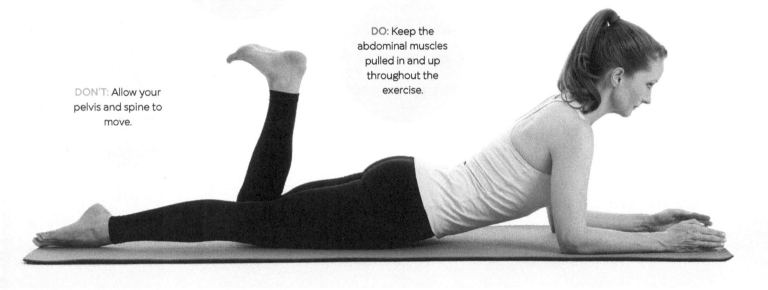

C   D   E

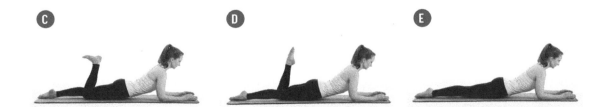

NECK PULL, MODIFIED

The Neck Pull is Pilates's way of making the Roll-Up (page 82) more difficult. The full Neck Pull is an advanced exercise that starts on your back with your arms behind your head, which increases the weight of the torso and makes the exercise much more challenging. This modified version starts in a seated position, instead.

FOCUS: Maintain the smooth C-curve of the spine throughout the full movement.

REPETITIONS: 4 to 6

VISUALIZATION: To achieve a nice, even curve, imagine your abs are the inside of an ice cream scoop and your back is the outside of the scoop.

PRECAUTIONS: If you have lower-back or hip flexor pain, you may need to modify the range of motion or perform the exercise with your hips higher than your feet. Individuals with a history of herniated discs should avoid the exercise.

1. Sit tall with your weight even on your sit bones, your pelvis neutral, your legs shoulder-width apart, and your knees bent with your feet flat on the floor. Place your hands behind your head at the base of your skull with your elbows reaching wide to keep the shoulders open. **A**

2. Inhale to pull your belly button to your spine.

3. Exhale to contract the abdominal muscles and roll back off your sit bones, scooping in your abs. **B** Continue to roll back as far as you can while still maintaining flat abs and a curved spine. **C** (However, if your bottom rib touches the mat, pause in that position.) The goal is to achieve a C-curve of the spine.

4. At your end range, inhale and focus on flattening your abs and keeping your wings down.

5. Exhale, maintain the C-curve, and roll forward until you arrive back on your sit bones with your spine curled over your knees. **D** **E**

6. From that position, inhale to roll up, one vertebra at a time, to return to the start position. **F**

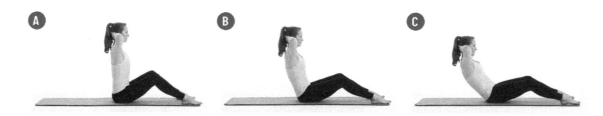

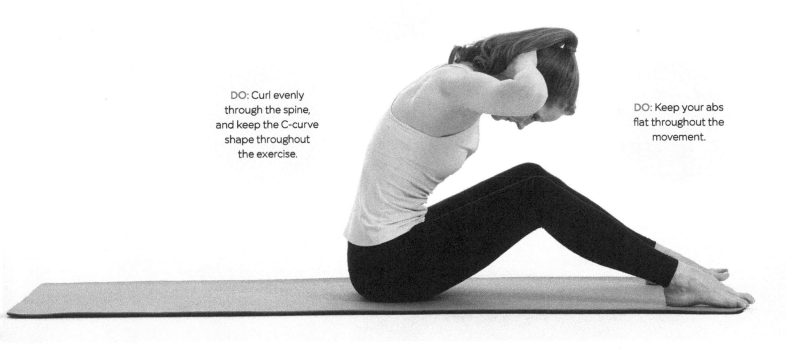

DON'T: Allow the shoulders to shrug.

DO: Curl evenly through the spine, and keep the C-curve shape throughout the exercise.

DO: Keep your abs flat throughout the movement.

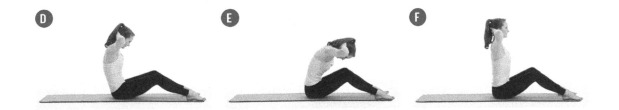

D

E

F

SIDE KICK SERIES

CIRCLES

The Circles exercise challenges the stability of the pelvis and the spine against the movement of the legs as the muscles around the leg work to control the movement.

FOCUS: Keep the spine, pelvis, and hips neutral as the top leg circles both forward and back.

REPETITIONS: 6 to 10 in each direction, on each side

VISUALIZATION: Imagine that your spine is a steel rod, impervious to movement, regardless of what the legs do. Imagine you have a pencil attached to your toes and are drawing small circles on the wall.

PRECAUTIONS: If you have a tight lower back, you may need to flex the hips slightly. Individuals with neck pain might need to place a pillow under their head.

1. Lie on one side with your hips stacked and your feet in line with your hips. Your body will be in a straight line. Extend your bottom arm overhead and allow your head to rest on it, or if it is more comfortable, bend your bottom arm and rest your head in your hand. Your top arm should be bent, with your hand resting on the floor. Make sure your pelvis and spine are neutral. **A**

2. Inhale to lengthen through the spine and pull your belly button to your spine, simultaneously lifting the top leg higher than hip height but keeping the knee facing forward. **B**

3. Circle the leg forward in very small circles, exhaling each time the top ankle passes by the other ankle, and taking a small sip of air at the top of each circle. **C** **D** **E**

4. After you've traced 6 to 10 circles, reverse the direction and trace 6 to 10 more very small circles with the same leg, exhaling each time the top ankle passes by the other ankle, and taking a small sip of air at the top of each circle.

5. Exhale and lower the leg down to the start position. **F**

6. Repeat on the other side.

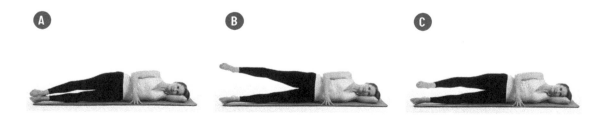

A   **B**   **C**

DO: Keep your abs
flat and your legs
engaged.

DO: Keep both knees
pointing straight
forward.

DON'T: Allow the
top hip to hike up
as the leg lifts.

DON'T: Put pressure
on your top hand or
let the shoulder roll
forward.

DON'T: Allow the
pelvis to rotate or
wobble as the leg
circles.

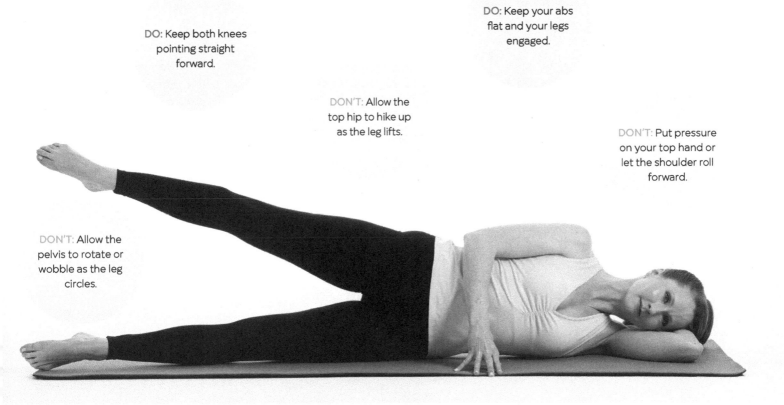

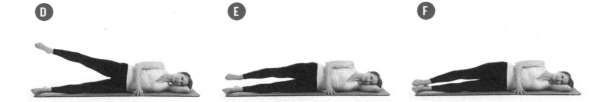

D   E   F

STAGGERED LEGS

This move capitalizes on the strength developed in the Up & Down (page 102) and Circles (page 128) exercises, demanding more stability of the pelvis and torso and more strength in the muscles of the hips and legs.

FOCUS: Keep the spine, pelvis, and hips neutral against the movement of the legs.

REPETITIONS: 4 to 6 on each side

VISUALIZATION: Imagine that your spine is a steel rod, impervious to movement regardless of what the legs do.

PRECAUTIONS: If you have a tight lower back, you may need to flex the hips slightly. Individuals with neck pain might need to place a pillow under their head.

1. Lie on one side with your hips stacked and your feet in line with your hips. Your body will be in a straight line. Extend your bottom arm overhead and allow your head to rest on it, or if it is more comfortable, bend your bottom arm and rest your head in your hand. The top arm should be bent, with the hand resting on the floor. Make sure that your pelvis and spine are neutral. **A**

2. Inhale to lengthen through the spine and pull your belly button to your spine, simultaneously lifting the top leg higher than hip height but keeping the knee facing forward. **B**

3. As you exhale, lift the bottom leg to meet the top leg. **C** Then, on that same exhale, lower both the legs down to the mat together. **D** Repeat 4 to 6 times.

4. Repeat on the other side.

A

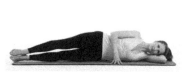

DO: Keep both knees pointing straight forward.

DON'T: Let the top leg drop. Keep it lifted and make the bottom leg meet it.

DO: Keep your abs flat and your legs engaged.

DON'T: Put pressure on your top hand or let the shoulder roll forward.

DON'T: Allow the top hip to hike up towards the ribs.

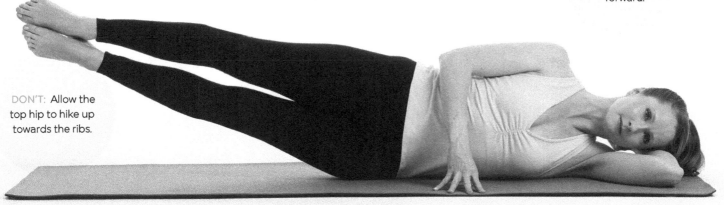

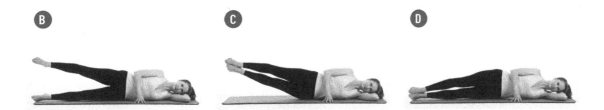

B

C

D

DOUBLE-LEG LIFT

The Double-Leg Lift is the culmination of all the Side Kick Series exercises. It works to strengthen the muscles of the outer hip and leg while stabilizing the spine and flattening the abs.

FOCUS: Keep the spine, pelvis, and hips neutral against the movement of the legs.

REPETITIONS: 4 to 6 on each side

VISUALIZATION: Imagine that your spine is still a steel rod, but now someone has sewn the inseam of your pants together so your legs cannot separate.

PRECAUTIONS: If you have a tight lower back, you may need to flex the hips slightly. Individuals with neck pain might need to place a pillow under their head.

1. Lie on one side with your hips stacked and your feet in line with your hips. Your body will be in a straight line. Extend your bottom arm overhead and allow your head to rest on it, or if it is more comfortable, bend your bottom arm and rest your head in your hand. Your top arm should be bent, with your hand resting on the floor. Make sure your pelvis and spine are neutral. **A**

2. Inhale to lengthen through the spine and pull your belly button to your spine.

3. As you exhale, lift both legs simultaneously, keeping the hips neutral, abs flat, and legs connected. **B**

4. Inhale as you lower both legs to the start position. **C** Repeat 4 to 6 times.

5. Repeat on the other side.

DO: Keep both knees
pointing straight
forward.

DO: Keep your
abs flat and your
legs engaged and
squeezed tightly
together.

DON'T: Allow your
legs to move forward
as they lift.

DON'T: Let the top
hip hike up towards
the ribs.

DON'T: Put pressure
on your top hand or
let the shoulder roll
forward.

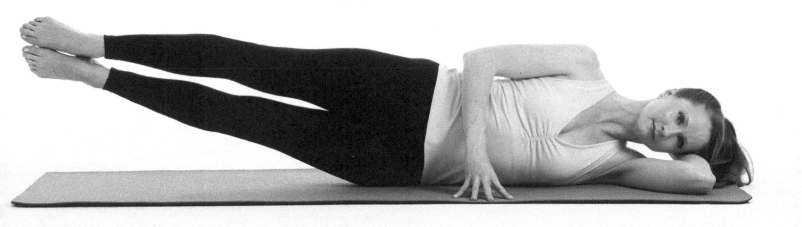

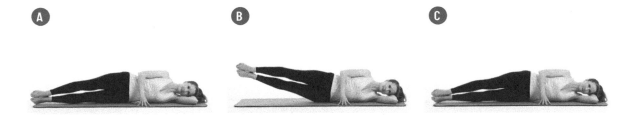

Ⓐ   Ⓑ   Ⓒ

THE TEASER, MODIFIED

This move builds on the strength and flexibility gained in the Roll-Up (page 82) and Open-Leg Rocker (page 116) by adding the challenge of rolling up with one leg straightened on a high diagonal. It improves abdominal strength, balance, and core control.

FOCUS: Roll smoothly up to the Teaser position without using momentum or moving the legs in space.

REPETITIONS: 4 to 6

VISUALIZATION: Imagine peeling a piece of tape off the mat slowly as the spine rolls up. Imagine placing a string of pearls down on a bureau, one pearl at a time, when rolling down. Envision your legs fixed in space on the high diagonal and that the spine must roll up to meet them.

PRECAUTIONS: If you've been advised to avoid rotation due to lower-back or disc injuries, skip this exercise until you are cleared by a medical professional. Always work in a pain-free range of motion. If you have a neck injury or neck pain, you may need to modify or skip this exercise.

1. Lie on the mat with both knees bent and feet flat on the floor, legs squeezing together, and your arms by your sides. **A** Move to the imprint position. Inhale and lift one leg up into a tabletop position. Then, extend that leg into a high diagonal, about 45 to 60 degrees off the ground. **B** Reach your arms overhead as far as possible, keeping your bottom ribs on the mat. **C**

2. Inhale smoothly and reach your arms to the ceiling, then lift your head and shoulders to start rolling up. **D**

3. On a strong exhale, continue rolling up, one vertebra at a time, reaching your arms toward your knees until half of your body is holding the Teaser position (like a V) with your weight on the back of your sit bones. **E**

4. Inhale smoothly, lift your arms overhead by your ears, and lengthen the upper back and neck, bringing them into their natural, neutral position. **F**

5. Exhale, keeping the leg still in space. Round the spine to roll the torso down to the mat, one vertebra at a time. **G** At the end of the exhale, reach your arms overhead. **H**

6. Repeat on the other side.

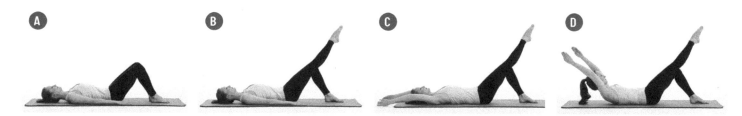

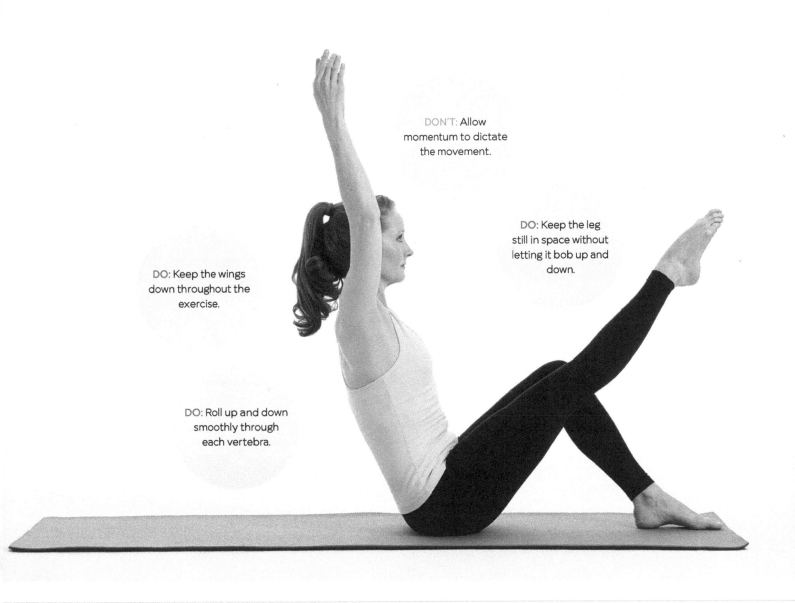

DON'T: Allow momentum to dictate the movement.

DO: Keep the leg still in space without letting it bob up and down.

DO: Keep the wings down throughout the exercise.

DO: Roll up and down smoothly through each vertebra.

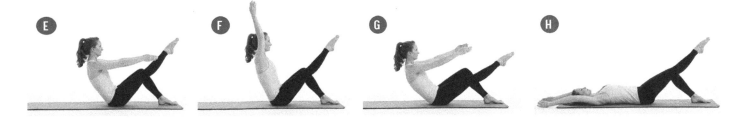

E

F

G

H

SWIMMING, MODIFIED

Swimming is an advanced exercise designed to strengthen the back and butt muscles and tone the upper arms. In this modified version, we help you start slowly to learn proper technique and execution for maximum benefit as you pick up the pace.

FOCUS: Lift your head, shoulders, and opposite arm and leg without bending your knee or overextending your neck.

REPETITIONS: 8 to 10 on each side

VISUALIZATION: Instead of thinking of lifting the opposite arm and leg, imagine the body getting longer with each repetition, as if you are the rope in a tug-of-war, being pulled from both ends.

PRECAUTIONS: If you've been advised against back bending (extension of the spine), be sure to limit extension and support this position with your abdominal muscles. Individuals with excessive lordosis of the lumbar spine may need to place a cushion under their hip bones or skip the exercise completely. Similarly, individuals with neck injuries or neck pain may need to avoid this exercise.

1. Lie on your stomach with your legs straight, separated and slightly rotated outward, with your toes pointed. Reach your arms overhead, slightly wider than shoulder-width apart. **A** Engage your abdominal muscles to lift your abs off the mat, lengthen your neck and spine, and slide your shoulders down your back.

2. Exhale smoothly and engage the back muscles to lift your head and shoulders off the mat, simultaneously lifting the right arm and left leg off the mat. Use your left arm for additional support, if necessary. **B**

3. Inhale smoothly and lower your head, shoulders, arm, and leg back to the mat, thinking of length. **C**

4. Exhale smoothly, and repeat the movement on the other side, lifting the right leg and left arm along with the head and shoulders. **D**

A

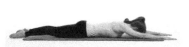

DON'T:
Hyperextend
your neck.

DO: Keep the neck
neutral and in line
with the rest of
the spine.

DO: Keep the legs
straight.

DO: Keep the abs
engaged throughout
the entire exercise.

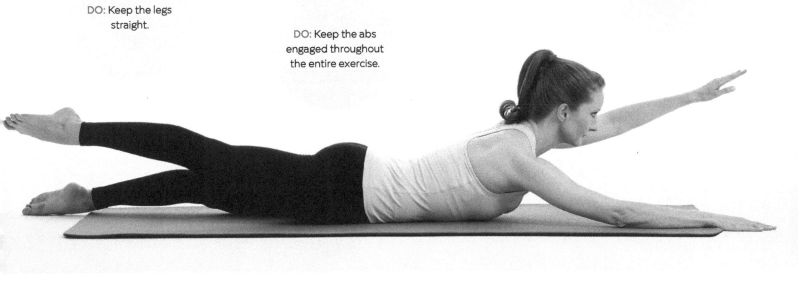

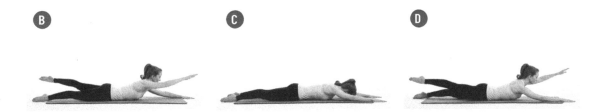

B   C   D

THE SEAL

The Seal builds on the strength gained in Rolling Like a Ball (page 86) by adding a balance pose at both ends of the movement (which challenges abdominal strength and core control). Plus, it's fun!

FOCUS: Maintain the C-curve of the spine. Balance at both ends of the movement to achieve 3 claps of the feet.

REPETITIONS: 6 to 8

VISUALIZATION: Imagine sitting as the letter C.

PRECAUTIONS: If you've been advised to avoid rotation due to lower-back or disc injuries, skip this exercise until you are cleared by a medical professional. Always work in a pain-free range of motion.

1. Sit tall with your weight even on both sit bones, your pelvis neutral, knees bent, legs squeezing together, and feet flat on the mat. **A** Contract the abdominal muscles to curve the spine and roll your weight back off the sit bones, gazing at your knees. **B** Then, lift your legs one at time and hold your ankles to balance on the back of your sit bones. Point the toes. **C** While maintaining balance, open your knees and slightly rotate your femurs out, keeping your toes together. Hold your ankles from the insides of your legs. This is the start position. **D**

2. Inhale smoothly and contract the abdominals to roll back to the top of the shoulder blades, but not onto your neck or head. Pause here long enough to clap your feet together 3 times. **E**

3. Exhale smoothly and contract the abdominal muscles more to slide the ribs toward the pelvis and return to the start position; balance here without putting the feet down, and clap the feet together 3 times. Repeat. **F**

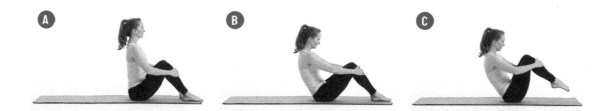

DON'T: Roll onto the
neck and head.

DO: Use the
abdominal muscles
as your brake and
accelerator.

DON'T: Allow
momentum to dictate
the movement.

DO: Keep your
wings down and
your neck long.

DO: Keep your
feet off the ground
in the start position
and between
repetitions.

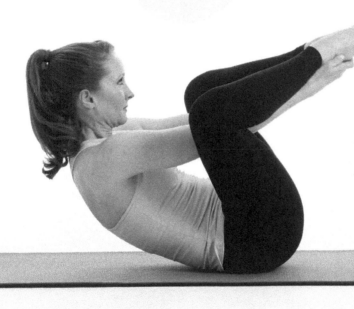

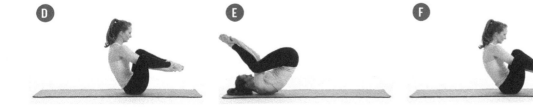

D   **E**   **F**

ASSESSING YOUR PROGRESS

Congratulations—you are no longer a Pilates beginner! After completing Level 2, you should feel gains in strength all over the body, improved posture, and increased confidence. Moreover, you should now have the body awareness to naturally incorporate Pilates principles into your daily life and other physical activities.

Here are some final assessment questions. If you still need work in any of these areas, continue with the Level 2 Program for one or two more weeks.

1. Can you perform the Level 2 exercises without any pain or discomfort?

2. Can you recognize any patterns of which exercises are easy or hard for you?

3. Are you able to reduce the range of motion to accommodate your unique needs?

If you answered "yes" to all three questions, we hope that you will continue on your Pilates journey, whether at a studio, a gym, or at home. If you like our style, then check out PilatesOnFifthOnline.com for more of our exercises!

We also include some supplemental strengthening exercises in the next chapter.

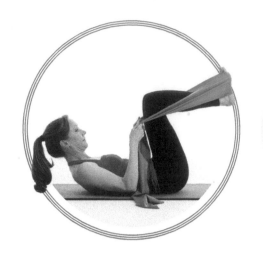

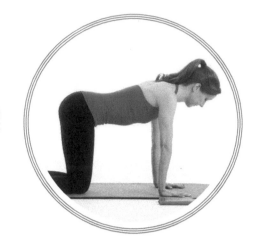

CHAPTER  7

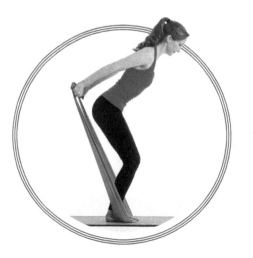

SUPPLEMENTAL STRENGTHENING EXERCISES

THE EXERCISES IN THIS CHAPTER are not in the traditional Pilates repertoire, but they are fabulous for building core strength quickly. These exercises can be performed at any time during your journey with this book, as they are great supplements for every program and level. Three of them call for a stretch band, which simulates the spring resistance Joseph Pilates used in the exercise equipment he invented. Stretch bands, like springs, require control throughout the exercise and thus tone the full length of the muscles. You can adjust where you hold the band to make easy adjustments in tension (difficulty).

ELBOW PLANK

An elbow plank builds core strength powerfully and effectively by targeting not just the abdominal muscles but also most of the muscles that compose your powerhouse. You'll achieve a strong core, sculpted arms, flat abs, and toned hips and thighs with this simple but challenging exercise.

FOCUS: Pull in your abdominal muscles tightly and protect your core with a neutral spine and pelvis.

REPETITIONS: Hold for 30 seconds, then 1 minute, then 1 minute and 30 seconds, and so on, up to 3 minutes. If you can hold your body in one straight line from the shoulders to the heels for 30 seconds without your back arching or aching, you may begin to try and hold the pose longer. If you feel your back arching or aching, however, put your knees down!

VISUALIZATION: Imagine that your body is an arrow, a straight line of energy starting at your heels and exiting out the top of your head.

PRECAUTIONS: If you have an exaggerated arch in your lower back, you'll need to build strength gradually. Start by holding the position only as long as you can maintain flat abs, a neutral spine, and a neutral pelvis. Build slowly from there.

1. From an all-fours position (page 17), place both your elbows on the mat directly underneath your shoulders. **A** Stretch one leg, **B** then the other, out behind you with your toes tucked, to form one straight line. Pull your belly button to your spine, squeeze your legs together, and engage your glutes. **C**

2. Inhale and exhale smoothly, holding this position for as long as you can maintain proper form.

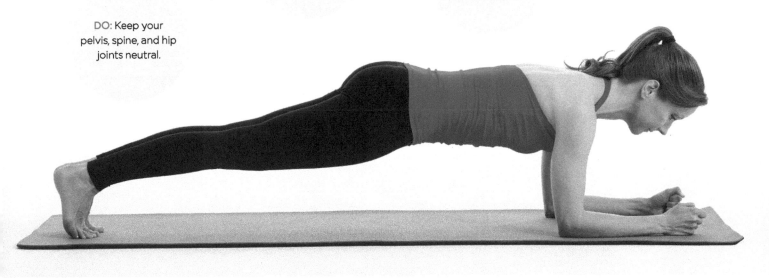

DON'T: Let your head fall toward the mat.

DO: Keep your belly button pulled in to your spine.

DO: Keep your body in a straight line from the heels to the shoulders.

DO: Keep your pelvis, spine, and hip joints neutral.

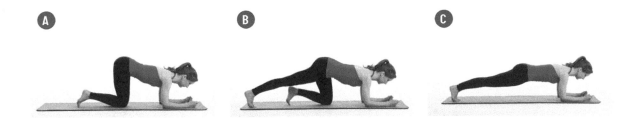

Ⓐ Ⓑ Ⓒ

SIDE PLANK

The Side Plank builds on the Elbow Plank by further challenging the serratus anterior, the gluteus medius, and the oblique abdominal muscles to hold the side plank position. Moreover, because most individuals tend to favor one side over the other, the side plank can be a great exercise to highlight and correct this imbalance.

FOCUS: For the duration of the exercise, keep your supporting shoulder strong and hips lifted to maintain a neutral spine and pelvis.

REPETITIONS: Hold for as little as 15 seconds or up to 1 minute per side

VISUALIZATION: Imagine a straight line drawn from the middle of your ankles to your ear.

PRECAUTIONS: If you're prone to neck pain, you may need to start with a very short hold of this pose, or skip it altogether. Similarly, individuals with shoulder injuries may need to reduce the hold time of the position or perform the exercise on their knees to lessen the burden on their shoulders.

1. Lie on one side with your hips stacked, and place your bottom elbow directly underneath your shoulder, propping your weight on the elbow. Make sure your hips are in line with your elbow and your feet are in line with your hips. Both legs should be straight, with your knees, hip bones, and shoulders facing forward. **A**

2. Inhale to prepare.

3. Exhale and press into your elbow and bottom foot to lift your hips off the mat, creating a neutral pelvis and spine and forming a straight line from your ankles to your ears. **B**

4. Continue to inhale and exhale smoothly, holding the position for as long as you can maintain proper form. Slowly increase your hold time as you build strength.

5. Repeat on the other side.

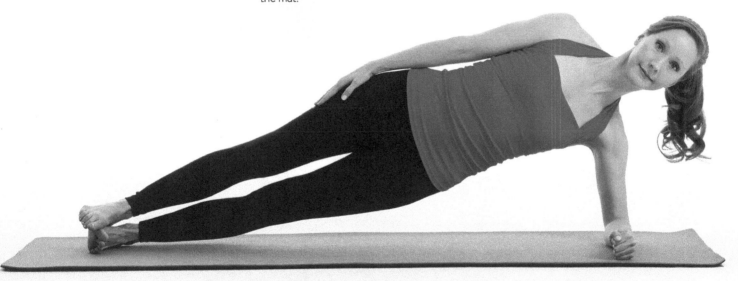

DON'T: Allow your hips to drop toward the mat.

DO: Keep your wings down and your neck long and neutral.

DON'T: Sink into your supporting shoulder.

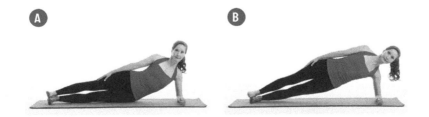

A

B

STANDING ARMS WITH STRETCH BAND

We've included varying versions of this exercise to target the different muscles in your shoulders and arms to give you strong, sculpted arms and more shapely shoulders!

FOCUS: Feel your arm muscles working without compromising your posture or feeling any strain in the neck.

REPETITIONS: 10 to 20 of each exercise

VISUALIZATION: Imagine the entire length of your arm muscles toning in the same way that a spring coil evenly disperses stretch and tension.

PRECAUTIONS: If you feel strain in the shoulder or elbow joints, adjust the tension as necessary.

1. Stand in the middle of the band with your feet sit-bones distance apart and grab the ends with your fists so the edge of the band is coming out the thumb side of your hands. Make sure your pelvis and spine are neutral and your wings are down. Pull your abdominal muscles in to your spine. **A**

2. For Biceps: Exhale and bend both elbows to bring your fists to your shoulders, keeping the upper arms in line with your torso. Inhale, straighten both arms, and return to the start position. Repeat. **B**

3. For Anterior Deltoids: Exhale and reach both arms forward to shoulder height or slightly higher. Inhale and lower both arms to the start position. Repeat. **C**

4. For Middle Deltoids: Exhale and reach both arms out to your sides, keeping your thumbs facing the ceiling. Inhale and lower both arms to the start position. Repeat. **D**

5. For Posterior Deltoids: Exhale and reach both arms back behind your torso, keeping your arms straight. Inhale and return to the start position. Repeat. **E**

6. For Triceps: Bend both elbows, pulling your fists up next to your ribs so the elbows are pointing directly back. **F** Keeping the upper arms fixed in space, exhale and extend the elbows fully to target the triceps. **G** Inhale and slowly bend the elbows to return to the previous position. Repeat.

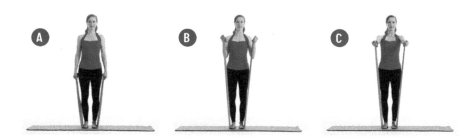

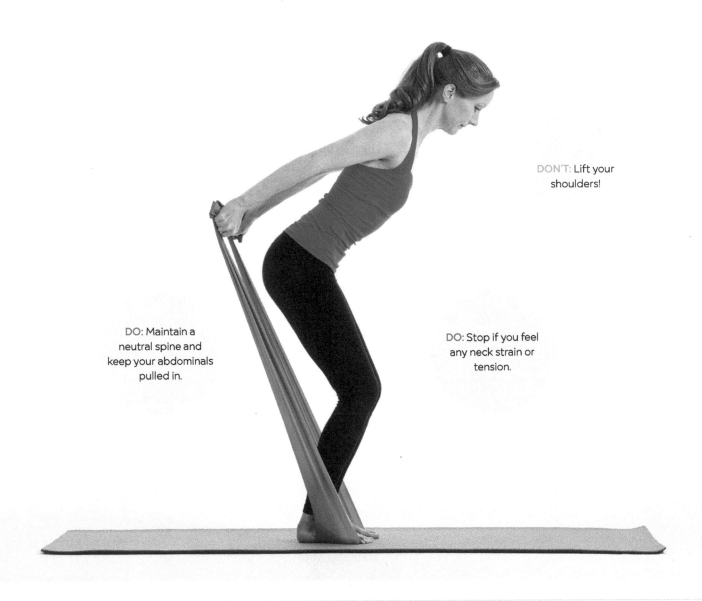

DON'T: Lift your shoulders!

DO: Maintain a neutral spine and keep your abdominals pulled in.

DO: Stop if you feel any neck strain or tension.

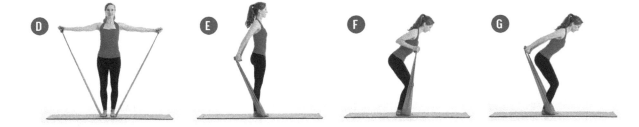

D   E   F   G

BEND & STRETCH WITH STRETCH BAND

During this exercise, the stretch band provides controlled resistance to strengthen and tone the muscles of the legs while targeting the abdominal muscles as well.

FOCUS: Extend the leg fully against the tension of the band while keeping the abdominal connection between the ribs and the hips and maintaining the imprint position.

REPETITIONS: 10 to 12 in each position

VISUALIZATION: With each repetition, imagine your legs are taffy being pulled, getting longer each time they are pulled.

PRECAUTIONS: If you have instability in your lower back, extend your legs on a higher diagonal to protect it. Be careful to keep tension out of your neck.

1. Lie on your back on the mat with your knees bent and feet flat on the floor, lower-back pressed into an imprint and abdominal muscles engaged. **A** Lift your legs up one at a time to tabletop position with your knees bent at right angles, and inner thighs squeezing together. **B** Take the band, curl your head and shoulders off the mat, and wrap the center of the band around the bottoms of your feet. Keep your feet flexed. Hold the edges of the band with your fists, with the band coming out the thumb side of your hands. **C** Relax your head and shoulders back down to the mat and slide the band through the hands to the desired tension. Bend your elbows so your fists point to the ceiling, and press your elbows and the backs of your shoulders into the mat. **D**

2. Parallel: Exhale, keep squeezing the inner thighs together, pull the abdominal muscles in, and extend the legs on a high diagonal against the tension of the band without moving your arms. **E** Inhale and bend the knees to return to the previous position. **F** Repeat.

3. Turned Out: Maintain the position of the body and band, but now, from the Parallel leg position, **F** keep your heels together and open the knees so your legs form a diamond shape. Your heels should be together and your toes apart, with the band still around the arches of the feet. Exhale, pull the abdominal muscles in, squeeze your heels together, and press your feet into the band to straighten your legs into a high diagonal without moving your arms. **G** Inhale and bend the knees to return to the previous position. Repeat.

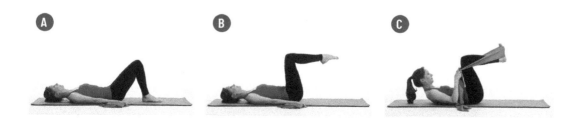

A **B** **C**

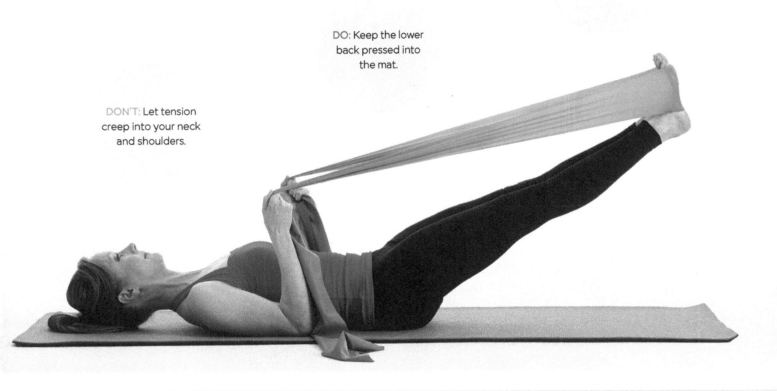

DO: Straighten the legs fully!

DO: Keep the lower back pressed into the mat.

DON'T: Let tension creep into your neck and shoulders.

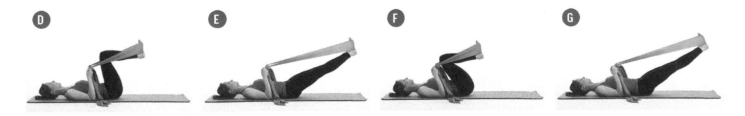

D   E   F   G

KICK BACK & KICK UP WITH STRETCH BAND

This move strengthens and tones the muscles in the backs of the legs, which can be difficult to "feel" in Pilates exercises (although they *are* working!). And, as a bonus, it also provides an instant feeling of a higher and tighter bum.

FOCUS: Strengthen the muscles of the buttocks and upper back of the leg without straining your lower back.

REPETITIONS: 8 to 10 of each exercise, on each leg

VISUALIZATION: As you kick your leg back or up, imagine your spine is a steel rod that cannot bend. For the Kick Up, imagine putting a footprint on the ceiling.

PRECAUTIONS: If you have instability in your lower back, limit your range of motion to ensure that the back does not arch during the exercises.

1. From an all-fours position (page 17), **A** reach the right foot forward and wrap the middle of the band around the arch of the foot. **B** While holding the ends of the band, return to the all-fours position. **C**

2. Kick Back: Exhale and press the right leg back against the tension of the band to extend straight and in line with the hip. **D** Inhale, bend the knee, and return to the previous position with your knee hovering for easy repetition. Do 8 to 10 reps, then carefully transfer the loop of the band to the left foot and repeat.

3. Kick Up: Keeping the knee bent at a 90-degree angle, lift the right leg back to extend the hip so the thigh is parallel to the floor and the foot is flexed and reaching to the ceiling. Exhale, hold the spine in neutral, and lift the thigh as if putting a footprint on the ceiling. **E** Inhale, and **F** lower slightly. Do 8 to 10 reps, then carefully transfer the loop of the band to the left foot and repeat.

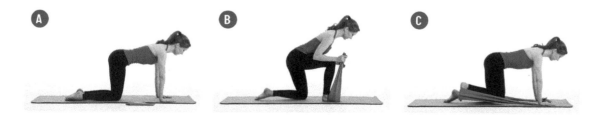

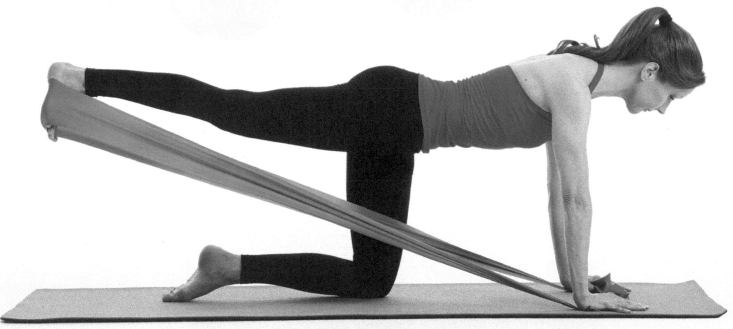

DON'T: Allow your spine to arch.

DO: Keep the abdominal muscles pulled in and your spine straight.

DO: Straighten the knee fully on the Kick Back.

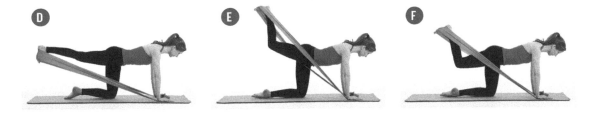

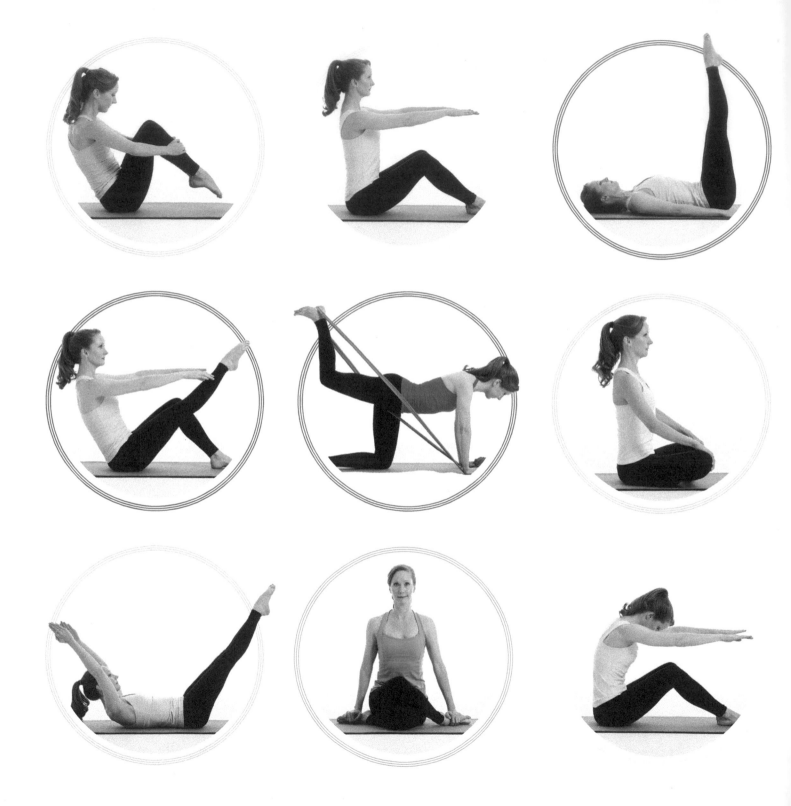

RESOURCES

TO LEARN MORE ABOUT PILATES, check out some of our favorite websites and publications:

For online video workouts, including step-by-step instructional videos to supplement this book, visit our website, PilatesOnFifthOnline.com. You will find workouts for all ages and fitness levels, as well as workout calendars to help you reach your goals. You can also visit our online shop to find some small equipment to supplement your mat Pilates practice.

Follow us on Facebook (Facebook.com/Pilates.On.Fifth) to connect with others in our Pilates on Fifth community, ask us questions, or make workout requests!

For research-based articles on the benefits of Pilates, visit the Pilates Method Alliance (PMA) website: PilatesMethodAlliance.org. Visit PMAShop.org to purchase books on Joseph Pilates and his original exercises.

To learn more about the history of Pilates, as well as get answers to frequently asked questions, we recommend MedicineNet.com/pilates/article.htm#what_is_the_origin_of_pilates.

For a fun Pilates community, visit PilatesStyle.com. *Pilates Style Magazine* is the only magazine dedicated to Pilates enthusiasts, and it is always full of great info!

Interested in learning more about Joseph Pilates and his original students? Meet Lolita San Miguel, at LolitaPilates.com, the only living person to have trained with Pilates himself and a mentor for many Pilates teachers.

For general fitness information, visit AceFitness.org.

INDEX

ACKNOWLEDGMENTS

TEACHING PILATES EFFECTIVELY DEMANDS MUCH more than a strong knowledge of anatomy, biomechanics, and, of course, the full repertoire of Pilates exercises. One must, above all, be an excellent teacher. Thus, we would like to acknowledge all the teachers we have had over the years—both academic and theatrical—who have helped make us the teachers we are today.

Our heartfelt thanks to Jane Kennedy, our former voice teacher, who is beautiful both inside and out, as she is the epitome of the skilled, compassionate teacher we both aspire to be.

Katherine would like to thank her husband, David Swirsky, for his unending love and support.

Many thanks to our Pilates teachers, including our first teacher, Candice Joseph, and our first certifying teachers, PJ O'Clair and Moira Stott Merrithew. We would like to thank our colleagues and mentors in movement: Lolita San Miguel, Kathy Corey, Mary Six Rupert, Joy Puleo and Balanced Body, Carrie Cohn, Amanda Iiams, Trent McEntire, Kimberly Dye, Alycea Ungaro, Shari Berkowitz, Linda Farrell, Connie Borho, Risa Sheppard, Amanda Altman, and Jonathan Hoffman.

Finally, as any labor-intensive small business owner knows, we depend on the skill and talent of our employees, and our teacher trainers and satellite centers worldwide. We sincerely thank all the employees and students we have had the pleasure to work with and train at Pilates on Fifth and Pilates Academy International over the years. We would not still be here without you!

ABOUT THE AUTHORS

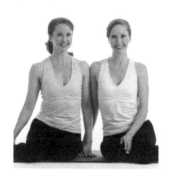

KATHERINE AND KIMBERLY CORP opened Pilates on Fifth in New York City 18 years ago after their practice of Pilates helped them transition from careers in corporate Japan to professional dancing careers with the Radio City Rockettes. Although they had danced since age three, the years of sitting through college, work, and then graduate school left them needing a solid, technique-driven exercise regime to "get their bodies back!" A fellow dancer recommended Pilates, and the two were soon hooked.

Katherine and Kimberly's diverse blend of experiences has equipped them with a unique understanding of both active and inactive people's needs. Thus, the pair is passionate about helping "regular people" reap the many benefits of Pilates. With this goal, they formed the Pilates Academy International, a Pilates teacher training program that now offers training at 45 satellite centers worldwide. To bring quality Pilates lessons to as many people as possible, Kimberly and Katherine created PilatesOnFifthOnline.com, an online streaming Pilates video website.

Katherine and Kimberly both hold bachelor's degrees in East Asian Studies from Duke University and master's degrees in International Economic Policy from Columbia University's School of International and Public Affairs. They hold personal training certifications from the American Council on Exercise (ACE) and the Pilates Method Alliance (PMA-CPT). To their great pleasure, Kimberly and Katherine still perform eye-high kicks with groups of former Rockettes, the Legacy Dancers and the Rockette Alumnae Dancers.

CPSIA information can be obtained
at www.ICGtesting.com
Printed in the USA
JSHW041826140323
38931JS00001B/1

9 781641 521505